The Mentor Connection in Nursing

ABOUT THE EDITORS

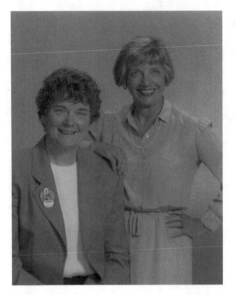

The editors: *(l. to r.)* Roberta K. Olson and Connie Vance.

Connie Vance, EdD, RN, FAAN, is Dean and Professor of Nursing at the College of New Rochelle School of Nursing, New Rochelle, New York, and a Fellow of the American Academy of Nursing. Her research and writing have been in the areas of mentorship, leadership development, and the professionalization of nursing. Dr. Vance holds an MSN in Psychiatric/Mental Health Nursing from Washington University, St. Louis, Missouri, and an EdD from Teachers College, Columbia University, New York, New York.

Roberta K. Olson, PhD, RN, is Dean and Professor of Nursing at South Dakota State University College of Nursing in Brookings, South Dakota. Her research and writing have been in the areas of mentorship, nursing education, and meta-analysis of nursing interventions and its effects on patient outcomes. Dr. Olson holds an MSN in Maternal-Child Health from Washington University, St. Louis, Missouri, and a PhD from Saint Louis University, St. Louis, Missouri.

The Mentor Connection in Nursing

Connie Vance
EdD, RN, FAAN

Roberta K. Olson
PhD, RN

Editors

 Springer Publishing Company

Copyright © 1998 by Springer Publishing Company, Inc.

Springer Publishing Company, Inc.
536 Broadway
New York, NY 10012–3955

Cover photograph from *Pueblo Stories and Storytellers* by Mark Bahti, 1988, Tucson, AZ:
Treasure Chest Publications, Inc. Reprinted with permission.
Cover design by Margaret Dunin
Acquisitions Editor: Ruth Chasek
Production Editor: T. Orrantia

99 00 01 02 / 5 4 3 2

Library of Congress Cataloging-in-Publication Data

The mentor connection in nursing / [edited by] Connie Vance. Roberta K. Olson.
   p.   cm.
   Includes bibliographical references and index.
   ISBN 0-8261-1174-2
   1. Mentoring in nursing. I. Vance, Connie. II. Olson, Roberta K.
   [DNLM: 1. Nursing. 2. Mentors. 3. Interprofessional Relations. WY 16
M519 1998]
RT86.45.M46 1998
610.73′06′99--dc21   97-41971
                                     CIP

Printed in the United States of America

On the cover: The Storyteller

Many of the pueblos of New Mexico and Arizona have a long-established tradition of clay figurines. The first contemporary storyteller figurine appeared in the mid-1960s when Helen Cordero of the Cochiti Pueblo expanded upon the mother and child figurines (sometimes called "singing mothers") and created a doll with many children (Bahti, 1988). The first storyteller doll she made was of a pueblo man with five children on his lap and shoulders, in memory of her grandfather, Santiago Quintana. Quintana, in the interest of maintaining and preserving his culture's traditions, worked with visiting anthropologists for over 40 years, beginning in the late 1800s. For even a longer period, he helped keep these traditions alive in the traditional manner of storytelling (Bahti, p. 7).

Ancient storytellers knew that tales are, in one of their oldest senses, a healing art. A story can be medicine which strengthens and guides the individual and community (Estes, 1992). Stories illuminate and give perspective to our lives, show us the best we can become, and provide clues on how to journey through life (Campbell, 1988). It has been suggested that we need to hear the stories of each other in order to appreciate the complexity and profundity of our lives and how to face the challenges that appear (Noble, 1990). Telling our stories can help us create new possibilities—for ourselves and for our profession. These narratives pass on the values and legacies of our profession and can assist us in composing new ways of being—as persons and as nurses.

Contents

Contributors   *xi*

Prologue and Message to the Reader   *xxi*

Acknowledgments   *xxv*

Part I: The Mentor Connection

1. Mentorship and Nursing   3

2. Mentoring for Career and Self-Development   11

   Mentor Remembered   19
     Anonymous

   Mentoring for Succession   25
     Margery Adams and Edward Beard, Jr.

   Reflections on Mentoring and Networks   32
     Geraldene Felton

3. Women Mentoring Women: Nurse to Nurse   35

   My Story about Women's and Nurses' Mentor Relationships   41
     Caroline M. Wright

Part II: Perspectives on Mentorship

4. Living the Mentor Connection: Personal
   Reflections and Stories   55

   Mentoring: A Song of Power   56
     Beverly Malone

   Interview of a Teacher-Mentor and Student-Protégé   60
     Jane K. Bruker and Melissa L. Charlie

   Mentorship: A Personal Perspective   66
     Marla E. Salmon

On Mentoring: A Skeptic's View   70
  Barbara Stevens Barnum

A Memorable Mentorship   75
  Virginia Trotter Betts

Tapping into Uncommon Wisdom through Mentorship   77
  JoEllen Koerner

A Leader's Mentors   83
  Clara L. Adams-Ender

Mentoring: An Interactive Process   87
  Ruth Watson Lubic

Full Circle: Peer Mentorship   89
  Caroline Erni and Susanne Greenblatt

The Privilege and Responsibility of Mentoring   93
  Hattie Bessent

Mentoring and Nursing's Relational Capacities   97
  Julie MacDonald

Mentoring Behaviors versus Mentoring Relationship: 100
  A Dissenter's Perspective
  Sandra K. Hanneman

Part III: The Process of Mentorship

5. Negotiating the Mentor Relationship   107

  The "Unintentional" Mentor   108
    Mary A. Cooke

  Mentorship in a Magnet Nursing Department   112
    Toni Fiore and Laura Cima

Part IV: Contexts for Mentoring

6. Mentoring in the Academic Setting   121

  Mentoring a Student—Growing a Leader   123
    Cynthia J. Rich Schmus

The Mentor Connection for Student Leaders   125
    Robert V. Piemonte

Mentoring Graduate Nursing Students in Home Health Nursing   127
    Felicitas A. dela Cruz, Lyvia M. Villegas, and Angeline M. Jacobs

Group as Mentor: Creating Academic Communities of Scholarly Caring
    Kathleen T. Heinrich   128

My Mentor   132
    Dianna P. Ross

My Role as Mentor   133
    Ventryce Thomas

The Mentor Program   134
    Lucia M. Rusty

Caring for Each Other: The Student and Alumni Mentor Connection 135
    Penny Bamford, Russell Hullstrung, and Mary Plitsas

A Model for Mentoring Junior Nursing Faculty   137
    Regina M. Sallee Williams

Reflections of Mentors: Nurse Leaders in Academe   139
    Mary Boose Walker

7. Mentoring in the Practice Setting   141

    The Head Nurse, Mentorship, Leadership, and Change   148
        Jane O'Malley

8. Mentoring for Scholarship and Research Development   151

    Mentors and Advances in Nursing Science   151
        Jacqueline Fawcett and Ruth McCorkle

    A Mentoring Circle: Facilitating Nursing Research with Staff Nurses
        Savina Schoenhofer and Mariamma Pyngolil   155

9. Group and Collective Mentorship   158

    Community and Health Professional Mentor Relationships   158
        Patricia Castiglia

    The Good Ol' Girls and Collective Mentoring   160
        Judith Kline Leavitt and Diana J. Mason

Executive Development and Mentorship   163
    Rachel Z. Booth, Geraldine (Polly) Bednash, and Michelle F. Pratt

Creating a Legacy of Leadership in the South   164
    Jean A. Kelley and Eula Aiken

Part V: Expanding the Mentor Connection

10. Global and Cross-Cultural Mentoring: Voices from the Field   171

Mentoring for International Educational Program Development   172
    Joyce J. Fitzpatrick

Global Mentoring: A Collaborative Process   176
    Carol Picard

The Hunter-Shanghai Project: An International Cross-Cultural   178
    Experience in Research Mentorship
    Evelynn C. Gioiella, Janet N. Natapoff,
    and Mary Anne N. McDermott

The New Zealand Midwifery Mentor Partnership   185
    Karen Guilliland

The Philippine Nurses' Network   188
    Marie F. Santiago

Mentoring Experiences at the Academy for Nursing Studies in India
    M. Prakasamma   192

A Study of Mentoring and Career Development of Directors of Nursing
    in South Australia
    Grant Sharples   196

Mentorship in Italy   199
    Renzo Zanotti

A Russian-American Tale of Mentoring   201
    Irina Ivancovich

Epilogue   205

References and Bibliography   209

Index   229

Contributors

Many persons contributed original stories, essays, and personal reflections on mentorship to this book. Some of these contributions are presented in their entirety, others are excerpts of longer pieces that could not be published because of space limitations. Together, they provide a mosaic of the different forms that mentorship takes in the nursing profession. Further, these reflections offer a multitude of perspectives on what mentorship has meant and can mean to individual nurses, students, and the profession. We are grateful for all of their voices.

KATHERINE ABRIAM-YAGO, EdD, RN
Assistant Professor
Student Retention Coordinator
School of Nursing
San Jose State University
San Jose, CA

MARGERY ADAMS, MN, RN, CNAA
Vice President Patient Services
Emerita, Catawba Memorial
    Hospital
Hickory, NC

CLARA L. ADAMS-ENDER, PhD (HON), RN, FAAN
Brigadier General
US Army (Retired);
President/CEO
CAPE Associates, Inc.
Lake Ridge, VA

EULA AIKEN, PhD
Project Codirector
Faculty Development for
    Graduate Nurse Educators
Executive Director
Southern Council on Collegiate
    Education for Nursing
Atlanta, GA

DEE BALDWIN, PhD, RN
Associate Professor
School of Nursing
Georgia State University
Atlanta, GA

PENNY BAMFORD, PhD, RN, CNAA
Associate Professor
School of Nursing
College of New Rochelle
New Rochelle, NY

**BARBARA STEVENS
BARNUM, PhD, RN, FAAN**
Professor
School of Nursing
Columbia University
New York, NY
Editor
Nursing Leadership Forum

**EDWARD BEARD, JR., MSN,
RN, CNAA**
Vice President, Patient Services
Catawba Memorial Hospital
Hickory, NC

**GERALDINE (POLLY)
BEDNASH, PhD, RN, FAAN**
Executive Director
American Association of
    Colleges of Nursing
Washington, DC

HATTIE BESSENT, EdD, RN
Emerita, Deputy Executive
Director
American Nurses Association
Minority Fellowship Program
Washington, DC

**VIRGINIA TROTTER BETTS,
JD, MSN, RN**
President
Health Futures, Inc.
Nashville, TN;
National Health Care Chair of
    Excellence
Professor of Nursing
Middle Tennessee State
    University
Murfreesboro, TN;
Immediate Past President
American Nurses Association
Washington, DC

RACHEL Z. BOOTH, PhD, RN
Dean and Professor
School of Nursing
University of Alabama at
    Birmingham
Birmingham, AL

JANE BRODY, PhD, RN
Assistant Professor
Department of Nursing
Nassau Community College
Garden City, NY

**DOROTHY BROOTEN, PhD,
RN, FAAN**
Associate Dean for Research and
    Graduate Studies;
John Burry, Jr., Professor of
    Nursing
Frances Payne Bolton School of
    Nursing
Case Western Reserve University
Cleveland, OH

JANE K. BRUKER, MSN, RNCS
Chair, Health Careers
Department of Nursing
University of New Mexico Gallup
Gallup, NM

CHERYL A. CAHILL, PhD, RN
Amelia Peabody Endowed
    Professor of Research
Institute of Health Professions
Massachusetts General Hospital
Boston, MA

**PATRICIA CASTIGLIA, PhD,
RNC, PNP, FAAN**
Dean
College of Nursing and Health
    Sciences
University of Texas at El Paso El
Paso, TX

MELISSA L. CHARLIE, MS, RN
Instructor
Nursing Program, University of
    New Mexico-Gallup
Gallup, NM
Doctoral Student
University of Pennsylvania
Philadelphia, PA

LAURA CIMA, MBA, CNA, CHE, RN
Director of Nursing
Surgical/Resource
Hackensack University Medical
    Center
Hackensack, NJ

ROSE ALLEN CLARK, DSN, RN
Professor
School of Nursing
Kentucky Wesleyan College
Owensboro, KY

MARY A. COOKE, MA, RN
Director
Cabrini Hospice
New York, NY

MARY COOPER, MS, RN
Nurse Manager
Johns Hopkins Hospital
Baltimore, MD

MARIA M. CVACH, MS, RN
Nurse Educator
Department of Medicine
Johns Hopkins Hospital
Baltimore, MD

NANCY DEBASIO, PhD, RN
Dean and Professor
Research College of Nursing
Rockhurst College
Kansas City, MO

FELICITAS A. dela CRUZ, DNSc, RN
Professor and Director
High Risk Home Health Nursing
Clinical Specialty and Family
    Nurse Practitioner Programs
School of Nursing
Azusa Pacific University
Azusa, CA

DORIS EDWARDS, EdD, RN
Dean and Professor
School of Nursing
Capital University
Columbus, OH

CAROLINE ERNI, BSN, RN
Case Manager
Emergency Department
St. Vincent's Medical Center
New York, NY

BARBARA A. FARLEY, MN, RN
Executive Director
Nursing and Patient Care
    Services
Medical College of Virginia
    Hospitals
Richmond, VA

JACQUELINE FAWCETT, PhD, FAAN
Professor
School of Nursing
University of Pennsylvania
Philadelphia, PA

GERALDENE FELTON, EdD, RN, FAAN
Kelting Family Professor of
    Nursing and Former Dean
College of Nursing
University of Iowa
Iowa City, IA

SUSAN BOWAR FERRES, PhD, RN, CNAA
Senior Administrator and
  Director of Nursing
Department of Nursing
New York Medical Center
New York, NY

TONI FIORE, MA, RN, CNAA
Vice President and Chief
  Nursing Officer
Hackensack University Medical
Center
Hackensack, NJ

JOYCE J. FITZPATRICK, PhD, RN, FAAN
Elizabeth Brooks Ford Professor
  and Dean of Nursing
Frances Payne Bolton School of
  Nursing
Case Western Reserve University
Cleveland, OH

KAREN E. FORBES, PhD, RN, CS, FNP-CS, CDE
Advanced Practice Nurse
Private Practice

HARRIET FORMAN, EdD, RN, CNAA
Executive Director
Nursing Spectrum
Ft. Lauderdale and Tampa, FL

RITA MUNLEY GALLAGHER, PhD, RN, C
Senior Policy Fellow
Department of Nursing
Practice, American Nurses
Association, Washington, DC

EVELYNN C. GIOIELLA, PhD, RN, FAAN
Dean and Professor
Hunter-Bellevue School of
  Nursing
Hunter College of the City
  University of New York
New York, NY

SUSANNE GREENBLATT, MAEd, RN
Case Manager
Emergency Department
St. Vincent's Hospital and
  Medical Center
New York, NY

KAREN GUILLILAND, RGON,
Advanced diploma in Nursing
National Director
New Zealand College of
  Midwives
Christchurch, New Zealand

SANDRA K. HANNEMAN, PhD, RN, FAAN
Associate Dean for Research and
  Evaluation
School of Nursing
University of Texas-Houston
Houston, TX

EILEEN HAYES, RNCS, FNP
Clinical Associate Professor
Co-Director
Primary Care Concentration
School of Nursing
University of Massachusetts
Amherst, MA;
Doctoral Candidate
University of Massachusetts

THORA HEESELER, MS, RN
Assistant Professor
Department of Nursing
Nassau Community College
Garden City, NY

KATHLEEN T. HEINRICH, PhD, RN
Associate Professor
Division of Nursing
University of Hartford
Hartford, CT

RUSSELL HULLSTRUNG, MPA
Administrative Coordinator
School of Nursing
College of New Rochelle
New Rochelle, NY

CAROL JORGENSEN HUSTON, MSN, RN, CNAA
Professor
School of Nursing
California State University
Chico, CA

IRINA IVANCOVICH, NURSE MIDWIFE
Director
Women's Health Promotion
Project
Saint Petersburg, Russia

ANGELINE M. JACOBS, MS, RN
Professor Emerita
Former Program Evaluator
High Risk Home Health Nursing
Clinical Specialty Program
School of Nursing
Azusa Pacific University
Azusa, CA

MARY ALICE JOHNSON, MS, RN
Director of Cardiovascular
Services
Union Memorial Hospital
Baltimore, MD

JEAN A. KELLEY, EdD, RN, FAAN
Project Co-Director
Faculty Development for
Graduate Nurse Educators
Professor Emerita
School of Nursing
University of Alabama
Birmingham
Birmingham, AL

JOELLEN KOERNER, PhD, RN, FAAN
Vice President for Patient
Services
Sioux Valley Hospital
Sioux Falls, SD
and Immediate Past President
American Organization of Nurse
Executives

LYNNETTE E. KRUEGER, MSN, RN
Psychiatric Nurse Clinician
Crisis Care Intervention
Danbury Hospital
Danbury, CT

DIANE R. LANCASTER, PhD, RN
Director
Nursing Research
Boston University Medical
Center
Boston, MA

ELAINE LARSON, PhD, RN
Dean
School of Nursing
Georgetown University
Washington, DC

**JUDITH KLINE LEAVITT,
MEd, RN, FAAN**
Generations United Director
Washington, DC

**RUTH WATSON LUBIC, EdD,
RN, CNM, FAAN, FACNM**
Expert Consultant
Office of Public Health and
    Science
US Department of Health and
    Human Services
Washington, DC

JULIE MACDONALD, MS, RN
Vice President
Patient Operations
Gundersen Lutheran Hospital La
Crosse, WI

BEVERLY MALONE, PhD, RN
President
American Nurses Association
Washington, DC;
Former Dean and Professor
School of Nursing
North Carolina A&T State
    University
Greensboro, NC

**DIANA J. MASON, PhD, RN,
C, FAAN**
Professor and Associate Dean for
    Graduate Studies
Lienhard School of Nursing Pace
University
New York City and Pleasantville
NY

**RUTH MCCORKLE, PhD,
FAAN**
Professor and Director
Center for Advanced Care in
    Serious Illness
School of Nursing
University of Pennsylvania
Philadelphia, PA

**MARY ANNE NELSON
MCDERMOTT, PhD, RN**
Associate Professor
Hunter-Bellevue School of
    Nursing
Hunter College of the City
    University of New York
New York, NY

AFAF MELEIS, PhD, RN, FAAN
Professor
School of Nursing
University of California
San Francisco, CA

ROSEANNA MILLS, PhD, RN
Chairperson
Department of Nursing
Nassau Community College
Garden City, NY

**JANET NIELSON NATAPOFF,
EdD, RN**
Professor
Hunter-Bellevue School of
    Nursing
Hunter College of the City
    University of New York
New York, NY

JANE O'MALLEY, RcpN, MA
Staff Nurse/Nurse Researcher
Acute Mental Health Services
Healthlink South
Christchurch
New Zealand
Doctoral Candidate
Victoria University of Wellington
Wellington, New Zealand

VALERIE PARKS, MS, RN
Nurse Manager
Department of Medicine
Johns Hopkins Hospital
Baltimore, MD

CAROL PICARD, MS, RN
Associate Professor
Department of Nursing
Fitchburg State College
Fitchburg, MA

ROBERT V. PIEMONTE, EdD, RN, FAAN
Former Executive Director
National Student Nurses'
    Association
New York, NY

MARY PLITSAS, BSN, RN
Research Nurse
Division of Medical Oncology
Columbia University
New York, NY

DOROTHY POWELL, EdD, RN, FAAN
Dean and Associate Professor
School of Nursing
Howard University
Washington, DC

M. PRAKASAMMA, PhD, RN
Professor
Academy for Nursing Studies
Hyderabad, India

MICHELLE F. PRATT, BA
Executive Assistant
Meeting and Membership
    Coordinator
American Association of
    Colleges of Nursing
Washington, DC

MARIAMMA PYNGOLIL, MSN, RN
Clinical Nurse Specialist
Broward General Medical Center
Ft. Lauderdale, FL

DIANNA P. ROSS
Alumna
School of Nursing
College of New Rochelle
New Rochelle, NY

LUCIA M. RUSTY, ACSW, CSW
Assistant Dean
Office of Student Services and
    Multicultural Affairs
School of Social Work
University of Maryland
Baltimore, MD
Former Director
Mentor Program
State University of New York at
    Stony Brook
Stony Brook, NY

MARLA E. SALMON, ScD, RN, FAAN
Associate Dean and Director of
   Graduate Studies
School of Nursing
University of Pennsylvania
Philadelphia, PA
Former Director
Division of Nursing
US Department of Health and
   Human Services
Washington, DC

MARIE F. SANTIAGO, EdD, RNC
Associate Profesor
School of Nursing
College of New Rochelle
New Rochelle, NY

CYNTHIA J. RICH SCHMUS, BSN, RN
Clinical Nurse
Oncology and Bone Marrow
   Transplant
Children's Hospital of
Philadelphia
Philadelphia, PA

SAVINA O. SCHOENHOFER, PhD, RN
Professor
Department of Graduate
   Nursing
Cora S. Balmat School of
   Nursing
Alcorn State University
Natchez, MS

GRANT SHARPLES, RN, RM, BEdN, MEd STUDIES
Clinical Coordinator
Whyalla Campus
School of Nursing
University of South Australia
South Australia

JUDY D. SHORT, DSN, RN
Associate Professor
Department of Baccalaureate
   and Graduate Nursing
Eastern Kentucky University
Richmond, KY

BARBARA M. STEWART, PhD, RN
Professor
Lienhard School of Nursing
Pace University
Pleasantville, NY

VENTRYCE THOMAS, MS, RN, CNA
Nursing Administrator for
   Clinical Affairs
University Hospital at
   Stonybrook
Stonybrook, NY

BERNADETTE VANDEUSEN, MSN, RN
Assistant Professor and Project
   Coordinator
Robert Wood Johnson Grant
Ohlone College Nursing
Department
Fremont, CA

LYVIA M. VILLEGAS, MA, RN
Former Recruitment
  Coordinator
High Risk Home Health Nursing
  Clinical Specialty Program
School of Nursing
Azusa Pacific University
Azusa, CA

**MARY BOOSE WALKER, EdD,
RN**
Assistant Dean for Graduate
Studies and Associate Professor
School of Nursing
Widener University
Chester, PA

**DIANA J. WEAVER, DNS, RN,
FAAN**
Senior Vice President, Patient
  Services
Yale-New Haven Hospital
New Haven, CT

**REGINA M. SALLEE
WILLIAMS, PhD, RN, FAAN**
Professor and Head
Department of Nursing
Education
Eastern Michigan University
Ypsilanti, MI

JUDITH WOLD, PhD, RN
Associate Professor
School of Nursing
Georgia State University
Atlanta, GA

**CAROLINE M. WRIGHT, PhD,
RN, CM**
Former Senior Lecturer
Postgraduate Coordinator
School of Health
University of Western Sydney
Richmond, NSW, Australia

**ROTHLYN P. ZAHOUREK, MS,
RN, CS**
Certified Clinical Specialist
Private Practice in Psychotherapy
Amherst, MA
Doctoral Candidate
New York University
New York, NY

CYNTHIA A. ZANE, EdD, RN
Dean
College of Health Professions
University of Detroit Mercy
Detroit, MI

RENZO ZANOTTI, PhD, RN
Professor of Nursing Theory
School of Nursing
University of Padova
Italy
Director of ISIRI (International
Institute of Nursing Research)

Prologue and Message
to the Reader

O ur journey to writing this book on mentorship has been a special adventure. Many fellow travelers have embarked on this journey with us through their studies, stories, and tough questions. As with any foray into the relatively unknown, there have been true believers and true skeptics. Both have enriched the exploration of mentoring and its ancient, contemporary, and futuristic dimensions. In the nursing profession, the first documented beginning of the journey began with Connie Vance's doctoral investigation at Teachers College, Columbia University, "A Group Profile of Contemporary Influentials in American Nursing," completed in 1977. At that same time, mentorship was gaining attention in diverse disciplines. Several landmark reports provided a foundation for intensive scrutiny of the mentor concept. Likewise, in the nursing profession, a flurry of empirical studies, opinion pieces, scholarly articles, and anecdotal reports provided evidence of the growing interest in mentoring. Roberta Olson completed her doctoral dissertation, "An Investigation of the Selection Process of Mentor-Protégé Relationships among Female Nurse Educators in College and University Settings in the Midwest," in 1984. Our interest in mentorship and its importance to the nursing profession fueled a collaboration that has extended over a decade—a partnership driven by a vision to inspire nurses about the need for mentoring each other.

Numerous investigators, including new and seasoned researchers and master's and doctoral students, consistently sought advice about instrumentation, bibliographies, and the location of mentoring work. There was obviously a line of research in mentorship being conducted, and we believed that information sharing and support were crucial in this effort. We began to collate data about mentoring studies in nursing across the country. Because much of the work at this point was fugitive and unknown, an extensive search process was used to locate these studies. During the period of 1977–1992, we located 81 nursing research studies on mentorship that were conducted in the United States and Canada. This compilation, *Mentorship in Nursing: A Collection of Research Abstracts with Selected Bibliographies*, was published in 1993. The research and writing on mentorship in our field has increased dramatically in the short period of 2 decades. There is a great desire to understand the concept and to activate it in the profession, as well as on behalf of the professional and leadership development of nursing students and nurses. The early literature and research focused on what mentoring is, whether it is present in the profession, and whether it is helpful or not. It can now be stated unequivocally that mentorship is a vital activity in our profession. The mentor connection in nursing is making an important contribution to the leadership and self-career development of students and practitioners. Continual questioning about a concept contributes to critical thinking, careful analysis, theory building, and sound research. We hope that this book will contribute to the ongoing dialogue about mentorship. At the same time, it should be understood that mentoring, like faith or love, is an elusive concept to define, "prove," and capture.

Mentoring is a complex human phenomenon that cannot be easily quantified. At the same time, we know mentoring when we see it or experience it. Its various definitional and theoretical formulations must be broadened to capture its richness, complexity, and diversity. Through qualitative studies and story telling, its presence, power, and influence in our lives may be shared and described but probably not elucidated fully.

We believe that strong mentor connections will continue to empower and expand our work as nurses and as caring women and men. We are convinced that even one kind and generous mentor can make a difference in another person's learning, growth and development. We are grateful for the community of believers both inside and outside the profession and for our network of colleagues and friends who live the mentor connection in spite of lingering obstacles. Everywhere we met and spoke with nurses, we found those who were enormously interested or deeply involved in mentoring at every career stage—from students to high-level leaders. Many were eager to share their experiences and ideas for developing and strengthening the mentor connection. We wish it were possible to include each of their perspectives—they were inspiring and deeply reflective of the great generosity and caring that nurses bring to their work with patients and with each other. Many of their stories are contained in this book. Many others will have to be told in different forums because of the space limitations of this book. It is our sincere hope that nurses' mentoring stories will continue to inspire us and to enrich our lives.

Acknowledgments

O ur collaboration has happily been more than the two of us. We are especially grateful to:

Special colleagues who generously shared their mentoring stories for this book. The scope of the book did not allow the inclusion of all of them. These narratives give expression to what has been unknown about mentorship in our profession. These stories are gifts of inspiration and show us the empowering nature of caring in the service of growth and learning.

Our faculty, staff, student colleagues, and friends who were important cheerleaders.

Dr. Ursula Springer, who believed in mentorship for the nursing profession from the beginning and encouraged us to tell the story. We also are thankful for the astute guidance and gentle encouragement provided by our editor, Ruth Chasek.

Members, colleagues, and staff of Sigma Theta Tau International, and many Chapters who provided numerous forums for the dissemination of the mentor concept in nursing across the country as well as internationally.

Our secretaries, Colleen Bimbo, Shirley Schliessmann, and Tara Anderson, who were true partners in the organization of the materials and for their many kindnesses.

Connie Vance also extends special gratitude to:

President Stephen Sweeny at the College of New Rochelle and Chancellor Dorothy Ann Kelly, O.S.U., who granted me an "at will" sabbatical to attend to "the muse."

The faculty, staff, and students of the College of New Rochelle

School of Nursing who were enormously supportive of my passion for mentorship and actualized the concept with each other.

The Sisters of St. Ursula, who provided kindness and peace at the Linwood Spiritual Center in Rhinebeck, New York. Their female community exemplifies the support and encouragement that women can give to each other.

Douglas Vance and Emily Vance, my children, for their graciousness and understanding of the necessity to spend long hours in the writing enterprise. Douglas kept my computer functioning, and Emily provided good cheer. I am forever thankful for the love and richness they bring to my life.

Roberta Olson especially thanks:

Dr. Carol J. Peterson, Vice President for Academic Affairs at South Dakota State University, who provided me with listening and time to reflect and write.

Drs. Penny Powers, Bill McBreen, Barbara Heater, and Judith Vinson, department heads at South Dakota State University College of Nursing, who provided support and reflection on mentoring.

David, Aaron, and Daniel Olson, my husband and sons, who gave me moral and emotional support to finish the writing and organizing that was essential for the final product.

PART I

The Mentor Connection

1

Mentorship and Nursing

Mentoring is a two-way circular dance that provides opportunities for us to experience both giving and receiving each other's gifts without limitations and fears (Huang & Lynch, 1995).

This is a book about a unique type of developmental relationship—the mentor connection. This connection is about colleagues helping each other grow and learn. It is a collegial connection that potentiates and empowers each person. Through these connections, professionals share information, teach each other, and strengthen the profession by ensuring an adequate supply of competent practitioners and leaders. These connections have been called "invisible colleges" because of their enduring educative effect (Moore, 1982). We believe that mentoring is essential to our full development as human beings and as professionals. It is possible, of course, to have a productive career without a significant mentor, but mentoring promotes career success faster and easier.

Mentor relationships have a profound impact on self and career development. Mentor relationships shape and nourish us. They have the capacity to transform the path of our human journey. The mentor-protégé relationship can be viewed as a gift-exchange phenomenon. "Its definition and the process by which it is discovered should be steeped in the vocabulary and the spirit of the gift . . . the definition should capture the giving and receiving, the awakening and the labor of gratitude. And finally, it should capture the passage to another that immortalizes the gift, and extends humankind. . . ." (Gehrke, 1988, p. 194). Mentoring also is an investment in the future. It is acting on a belief in the potential of our colleagues and students and implies a willingness to share the beauty of our dreams. Mentors give us hope—mentors believe in and nourish our dreams and expect us to reach for them. The "expectation effect" of mentoring plays a powerful role in our success and satisfaction. The voice of Dr. Harriet H. Werley, distinguished professor, author, administrator, and role model for research, expresses it: "As I look back on my life, I guess one of the things that always sustained me was the fact that people believed in me and expected me to do well, and I was treated accordingly. One of my mentors . . . is 95 years old now, and she is still my good friend and counselor" (Werley, 1988, p. 365). Mentoring creates and deepens connections that enrich both our personal and work lives. Success can be viewed as maximizing and developing the gifts and talents of others so that many will benefit (O'Neil, 1995). True mentoring creates this expanding spiral of success.

The centrality of mentoring to the developmental process of self and work has been acknowledged from the times of the ancient Greeks, Romans, and Chinese to the present. In the heroic age of Homer, Mentor was the trusted friend of Odysseus who was left in charge of the household and of his son during Odysseus's odyssey. An obscure twist to this legend is that it was Athena, the goddess of wisdom, who was disguised as Mentor and guided Odysseus's son, Telemachus, in the search for his father. In Greek mythology, Athena also appeared as Mentor to Hercules, giving him the golden apples gathered from the tree of life, thus guaranteeing him immortal status. Athena is depicted as lending support to Hercules by giving him special gifts that ensured his success, happiness, and immortality. Mentor—usually studied as a male phenomenon—is clearly manifest as a female goddess, serving as the protector, adviser, patron, and ally of heroic men (Bolen, 1985). These are intriguing clues to what being a mentor encompasses: a wise guide and protector, possessing androgynous behavior, who serves as an ally, supporter, and gift giver. In the spiritual tradition of Taoism in ancient China, the secrets of legendary leaders, kings, and rulers also were contained in the principles of mentoring. These were based on insights into human nature, leadership succession, teaching and learning, as well as giving and receiving wisdom in all relationships (Huang & Lynch, 1995). Historically, then, Mentor/Athena is an androgynous concept. A good mentor is intuitive, nurturing, objective, and directive. Mentoring is a harmony between the two poles of cosmic energy—the magical dance of opposites—natural components of one's total being (Huang & Lynch, 1995).

We believe that the mentor connection is a developmental,

empowering, and nurturing relationship extending over time in which mutual sharing, learning, and growth occur in an atmosphere of respect, collegiality, and affirmation. A mentor advises, guides, encourages, and inspires another person during an extended period of time. The mutuality inherent in the relationship means that all who enter it—those who mentor and those being mentored—will realize the many benefits of sharing and learning. Therefore, a mentor can be an advanced-level colleague or a peer-colleague. Mentoring is complex and elusive—difficult to define and to measure. It cannot be seen, but is a powerful, enriching phenomenon that can be described by those who experience it.

The colleague system, which includes mentoring, has always been present in the older established professions and in business. The predominance of these mentoring relationships was among men. Indeed, it was openly acknowledged that gaining entrée into the inner circle of leadership and moving up the professional and corporate success ladders entailed having a mentor. A landmark study of the developmental stages of men described the mentoring relationship as one of the most complex, and developmentally important a man can have in early adulthood (Levinson, Darrow, Klein, Levinson, & McKee, 1979). In another study of successful men, it was found that sustained relationships with loving people, such as mentors, produced the "best outcomes" in both their personal and career lives (Vaillant, 1977).

The issue of mentoring among women was not addressed until the late 1970s. It was acknowledged that there was a great need for career-oriented women to have mentors, and at the same time, it was acknowledged that it was often more difficult for them to find mentors. Connectedness, relationships, inclusion, and community always have been central values in women's lives (Belenky, Clinchy, Goldberger, & Tarule, 1986; Gilligan, 1993; Helgesen, 1990). Mentoring relationships, which encompass these elements, are a natural way for women to enhance their professional and work connections, as well as their teaching and learning and leadership development. A mentor's presence in a woman's career appears to be crucial at two periods—in the early phase and for the final push toward achieving leadership status—where still too few women venture and role models are scarce (Halcomb, 1979). Women also have begun to address the limitations of being mentored by men in the traditional framework. They are expanding the definitions and conception of the mentor relationship. It has been found that the male-mentor/female-protégé dyad frequently broke down when the woman got married, had children, and attempted to establish a balance between work and family life (Jeruchim & Shapiro, 1992). Only a female mentor can provide female role modeling and understand distinctive female challenges. A study of the relationship between mentoring and androgyny—an integration of masculine and feminine behaviors—suggested that a helpful mentor manifests androgynous behavior (Schoolcraft, 1986, 1995). Clearly, there is an evolving nature to the heretofore accepted parameters of mentoring.

In female-dominant professions, such as nursing, education, and social work, that are characterized as nurturing and helping disciplines, it might be expected that extensive mentoring of women by women would occur. In reality, however, even in these fields, mentoring has been underutilized. Are mentors needed in order to succeed in nursing? What is the effect of mentorship on professional development, clinical care, and scholarly productivity? These questions have been raised in the search for the role that mentorship can play in a largely female profession (Campbell-Heider, 1986; Hagerty, 1986; Jowers & Herr, 1990). Historically, many leaders in the field of nursing from Nightingale to today's leaders have experienced the benefits of having mentors (Fields, 1991; Schorr & Zimmerman, 1988). The first systematic investigation of mentor relationships among nursing leaders in the United States concluded that mentorship is an important source of influence among nursing leaders (Vance, 1977). Their mentor connections most likely contribute to the succession of leadership in the profession. These leaders' mentor relationships, however, showed divergence from the traditional model of mentoring. For example, in contrast to the one, all-encompassing mentor, multiple mentors characterized their relationships and provided a wide variety of mentoring assistance. Peer-colleagues and work supervisors were unusually important to them, and the majority of their mentors were women. It also appears that nurses at all levels benefit from mentoring assistance. An early study of mentor relationships between expert nurse clinicians and novice nurses reported that each person in these developmental relationships experienced work satisfaction, and quality patient care was enhanced (Atwood, 1979).

It has become increasingly evident that nursing, as a largely female profession, is a standard-bearer for women's issues, including mentorship. The profession provides a mirror of an evolving model of development and support for professional women that reflects the female experience and women's unique personal and career challenges. There is an emergent nature, almost a "work in progress," to the story of women mentoring women as they create different approaches to helping and supporting each other. It is our belief that women and nurses are inventing a new and evolving paradigm of mentorship. Women's and nurses' voices provide truths about the uniqueness of their mentoring experiences with each other. Through their stories they share and model new ways of enhancing each other's self and career journey. In the same way that women have placed their distinct marks on evolving models of growth, learning, and leading, they are defining and establishing new forms of mentoring. "As more women find our voices and demand to be heard, . . . we have an unprecedented opportunity to transform our planet with the values and skills we have honed over the centuries: caring, cooperation, community, and connection" (Noble, 1994, p. 197).

The "new mentorship" that has arisen out of a predominantly female profession—nursing—incorporates the essence of female values and skills. Through this emerging paradigm, we have an unprecedented opportunity to strengthen our identity as women and nurses and to create new models of support and achievement in our schools, workplaces, and the profession. The "new mentorship" suggests that students and teachers, novices and expert nurses, superiors and subordinates, and peer-colleagues can engage in a variety of growth activities among each other. Through a revisionist model of mentoring, the enhancement of identity and the creation of new support and success models can occur, as well as the establishment of different value systems. Perhaps we can thereby transform and humanize the professions, our schools, and our organizations. Perhaps we can rewrite some professional and organizational rules because of our unique mentor connections that will influence change and provide new emphases in our work and personal lives.

NATURE OF THE MENTOR RELATIONSHIP

Several theoretical frameworks provide a foundation for understanding the contribution of mentoring to human development. Erikson's stage of "generativity" (1963, 1968) is manifest by the human need to reach out to others to provide guidance and nurturance. Inherent in generativity is the acceptance of responsibility for passing on wisdom to the next generation. A mutually enriching experience for both the helper and the recipient is inherent in the relationship. The social learning theory of Bandura is another theoretical backdrop for mentoring

Success   **Satisfaction**
(Professional)   (Personal)

Professional   Self-Development
Development

FIGURE 1.1 Developmental outcomes of mentorship.

(1977). This theory is based on the imitation of modeling behavior of another. The value of learning through modeling, as compared to trial-and-error learning, is the acquisition of a larger, better integrated behavior pattern. Modeling is an inherent part of the mentor process throughout various stages of self and professional development. A third framework, provided by the study of on adult development in men and the importance of mentor relationships in realizing the "dream" (Levinson et al., 1979), was eventually extended to women. It was concluded that women experience similar stages of adult development, albeit with differences in "life circumstances, in life course, in ways of going through each developmental period" (Levinson, 1996, p. 36). It is clear that women address the developmental tasks of each stage with different experiences, resources, and constraints.

Regardless of which developmental approach is used in understanding the mentor concept, it is clear that there are two major developmental outcomes of mentoring to persons in a supportive mentoring relationship: success and satisfaction. These outcomes are depicted in Figure 1.1. Persons whose talents and abilities have been nurtured and promoted by caring mentors experience professional success easier and faster. They are better equipped to realize their "dream" and accomplish their goals as they move through various life and career stages. Future possibilities are articulated and doors are opened by the mentor's intentional assistance and guidance and by the mentor's belief in the protégé. Personal satisfaction and self-development are also promoted by the mentor relationship.

BENEFITS OF MENTORING

The two major developmental outcomes of success and satisfaction provide the background for viewing the specific benefits of mentor connections. These benefits accrue widely to both mentors and protégés, to the workplace, and to the profession. Analyses of stories, anecdotal accounts, self-reports, and qualitative studies suggest the following benefits of nurses' mentor connections:

1. Career success and advancement
2. Personal and professional satisfaction
3. Enhanced self-esteem and confidence
4. Preparation for leadership roles and succession
5. Strengthening of the profession

Both mentors and protégés experience greater *career success and advancement* because they are able to accomplish life-career goals easier and faster. Fewer mistakes are made. Dreams are encouraged, even if they are put on hold for periods of time. Long- and short-term career planning provides a road map for obtaining appropriate education and experience. *Personal and professional satisfaction* occurs through sharing of stories, insights, and experiences by mentor and protégé. This sharing is a mutual source of encouragement and modeling. Guidance and nurturance from a mentor enhance *self-esteem and self-confidence*. Self-analysis and increased self-assurance develop through honest sharing of insights and experiences. *Preparation for leadership roles and leadership succession* occurs through role modeling and rehearsal for new challenges. The "mentor is an honest mirror" (O'Neil, 1996) who provides feedback for risk taking in uncharted territory. Another important element of mentorship is the potential for "growing" leaders, thus *strengthening the profession* by ensuring continuity and quality leadership. There also is fun and joy in guiding each other through various stages of growth and development. Mentors and protégés report a sense of renewal as they are mutually stimulated to expand their skills and knowledge by each other's questions, specific challenges, and belief in one another.

To realize benefits of the mentor connection, there must be a willingness to give and to receive the precious gift of mentoring. Not everyone experiences the joy and pleasure of developing in relationship with a caring teacher-mentor or peer-mentor. In contrast, many long-distance leaders and winners treasure the company of mentor-friends and go to great efforts to cultivate these relationships (O'Neil, 1996). The nurse-influentials studied by Vance (1977) established and maintained their success and domain of influence through various personal, educational, and mentoring factors. They experienced the benefits of mentor connections throughout their careers. In nursing as well as in other disciplines, a chain of influence, consisting of influential leaders, their mentors, and their protégés, assists in ensuring continuity of leadership, professional socialization, and the growth and evolution of the profession.

2

Mentoring for Career and Self-Development

Mentors are suffused with magic and play a key part in our transformation. Their purpose . . . is to remind us that we can, indeed, survive the terror of the coming journey and undergo the transformation by moving through, not around, our fear. Mentors give us the magic that allows us to enter the darkness: a talisman to protect us from evil spells, a gem of wise advice, a map, and sometimes simply courage. But always the mentor appears near the outset of the journey as a helper, equipping us in some way for what is to come, a midwife to our dreams (Daloz, 1986).

The human journey of life and career has been described by various developmental models. These models provide a map that frames the setting for the journey and offers a context for growth and change. This human map "indicates landmarks, points out dangers, suggests possible routes and destinations" (Daloz, 1986). One of these maps is contained in the longitudinal study of the lives of 40 men in *The Seasons of a Man's Life* (Levinson, Darrow, Klein, Levinson, & Mckee,1978). A major contribution of this work was the emphasis on the role that mentors play during crucial life periods. A follow-up study, *The Seasons of a Woman's Life* (Levinson, 1996), reported that women and men go through the same sequence of life periods at the same ages, but also demonstrate wide variations between and within the genders, and in concrete ways of traversing these periods. "A

strongly male-centered view of adult life has for centuries been prevalent in our scientific and cultural institutions. It will take time, effort,
and sharpened awareness of gender issues to achieve a more balanced view [of women's development]" (Levinson, p. x). An alternative map of human development has evolved, based on the female
experience, in which connection and care are central, in contrast to
separateness and hierarchy (Gilligan, 1993). Because of diverse personal, family, and work commitments, women's life stages are characterized by improvisation, fluidity, diversity, and discontinuity
(Bateson, 1990). The complexities of contemporary society suggest
that lives of multiple commitments and multiple beginnings are an
emerging pattern rather than an aberration for many people.
Developmental maps that emphasize the interweaving of the individual with family and work, as well as spiral patterns of changing
careers and life events, provide a more accurate and holistic view of
contemporary human development.

One unifying theme of these life and career developmental models is clear: the acknowledgment of the central importance of helping
relationships, such as mentors and role models. The sustained, loving
involvement of various support persons in the life and career journey
of every human being is a necessity. Indeed, a person's life depends
(literally, in the first few years of life and in every other way in the
ensuing years) on whether someone is moved to care for us. "Our survival and development depend on our capacity to recruit the invested
attention of others to us" (Kegan, 1982, p. 17). It has been pointed out
that the need to nurture human growth should be a matter of concern
for our entire society, even more fundamental than sustaining productivity. "For all of us, continuing development depends on nurture and
guidance long after the years of formal education, just as it depends on
seeing others ahead on the road with whom it is possible to identify"
(Bateson, 1990, p. 55). This is especially true for those who have experienced barriers and various forms of discrimination that have created
self-doubt and diminished self-esteem. However, every human being
is at risk through all of life's unfolding experiences, which present new
problems and challenges and require concomitant change and new
learning. More than ever in a complex and turbulent world, we long
for kind and honest mentors who believe in, inspire, encourage, and
support us.

It is widely acknowledged that mentor relationships are essential
to professional socialization and to a fully developed career. It has
been demonstrated consistently that at each stage of a career, and

within each stage, some form of guided assistance is crucial for proper development. The complexity of a nursing career requires a substantial and consistent support system to ensure success and satisfaction. Mentoring partners provide assistance with the particular challenges and tasks inherent in each life and career stage—whether it be as student, neophyte nurse, clinician, teacher, researcher, manager, or administrative leader. Although career stages follow a somewhat predictable sequence in most career developmental models, mentoring relationships influence the form, quality, and outcome of the career path. For example, it appears that mentors are especially important at the beginning of one's career and at crucial turning points during that career. There will be periods when additional support is helpful, such as when assuming a new position or a new work role.

A review of the types of mentoring received by nurse-influentials in the Vance study (1977) as well as the factors they identified as critical to their career success and satisfaction was conducted. Based on the data, a paradigm has been developed that illustrates the types of mentor influences that were important to these nurse-influentials at each developmental stage. An adaptation of Super's model of vocational life stages (1957, 1963) provides a framework for viewing the prototypes of mentoring that the leaders received at each stage of their careers. The conceptual thrust of Super is that career development follows the principles and stages of human development and that career encompasses all roles in a lifetime. In other words, career and life development and role socialization is a continuous developmental process proceeding through specific life stages, from early childhood through adulthood. The life-career stages proposed by Super are: *growth* (birth–14 years); *exploration* (15–24 years); *establishment* (25–44 years); *maintenance* (45–64 years); and *decline* (age 65 and above). An expert panel reviewed these stages and the fit with the types of mentoring identified by the nurse-influentials. This panel found that the originally named stages in the Super model did not reflect appropriately the evolving nature of mentoring at each life-career stage. Therefore, these stages were renamed to convey a more dynamic picture of the life-career developmental process as it relates to mentoring. The renamed stages are: *education, exploration, expansion, establishment,* and *evolution.* The ages in each serve as approximations. Table 2.1 presents the paradigm of stages of life and career development and the types and descriptions of mentoring that are inherent at each stage.

The paradigm illustrates several points. First, the need for mentoring

TABLE 2.1 Paradigm of Life-Career Stages of Development and Types of Mentoring Help

Stages of Life-Career Development	Types of Mentoring Help Through Life Career
Education (Birth–14 years)	**Parent-Sponsor** Gender, role, and career identification Family and peer involvement, support, and guidance
Exploration (Age 15–24)	**Intellectual-Guide** Teaching, tutoring, counseling Expert advice and guidance Intellectual stimulation **Sociocultural role model** Introduction and socialization to society and profession
Expansion (Age 25–44)	**Visionary-Idealist** Believer in potential and dreams Establishes standards, expectations, and ideals Shaper of career **Promoter-Coach** Identifies options and resources Access and exposure to people and opportunities Career advisement and support
Establishment (Age 45–64)	**Peer-Colleague** Friendship, sharing, advice Confidant
Evolution (Age 65 and above)	**Mentor Emeritus** Recipient of friendship and recognition Satisfaction in generativity

Source. Super (1957, 1963). Adapted from Vance (1986). Copyright 1957, 1963, and 1986, respectively, by Harper, the Entrance Board, and Dissertation Abstracts International. Adapted with permission.

occurs throughout the entire self and career cycle. Second, self and career developmental stages are intertwined and require a variety of mentoring assistance at each stage. Third, the value of mentoring experiences arises from the developmental needs of the protégé at each developmental stage, as well as from the strengths and attributes of the mentor.

Who should assume the responsibility for the career development of the individual nurse? We suggest that this is a shared responsibility or partnership among the nurse, peers and advanced colleagues, the profession, and the organization. First, each nurse should be proactive in the development of her personal and professional growth and learning. She must demonstrate initiative, curiosity, a keen desire to learn, a career commitment, and actively seek the help of peers and experienced professionals. Second, seasoned professionals should be on the lookout for promising persons who desire to grow and expand their horizons and assume an active helping role in their development. It has been suggested that it is not evil or abusive people who derail or ruin careers, but rather the indifference of people who become so involved in their own work that they forget junior people (Hoffman, 1995). The profession and the workplace also exert considerable influence on the mentorship of new people in a discipline. Does the profession and the workplace have a demonstrated commitment to the development and support of neophytes? Are there formal mechanisms for promoting leadership development and succession? Are networking and sharing encouraged? The culture, values, and reward structures in work organizations either impede or encourage employees to develop their potential and to make a substantial contribution to the organization. It is clear that organizations demonstrate a great need for the benefits that can be realized from close, deliberate mentor relationships between seasoned employees and newcomers. The "learning organization" described by Senge (1990) emphasizes dialogue and support among people in an organization. He suggests that when a climate is established in which teams of people learn together—mentoring each other—the organization continually expands its capacity to create and to grow. Unfortunately, many bureaucratic organizations are still not structured to support this reality and to reap the benefits. "This is new work for most experienced managers, many of whom rose to the top because of their decision-making or problem-solving skills, not their skills in mentoring, coaching and helping others learn" (Senge, p. 345).

A growing number of studies provides empirical evidence that having a mentor is related to a protégé's achieving career success, often at an earlier age. This support is particularly important in the beginning of the career. In other words, mentoring can make a significant difference in career development in that one can achieve it easier and faster with the support of active, involved mentors. Mentoring relationships also provide the impetus and encouragement for obtaining advanced education and advanced positions. Mentoring is, therefore, an important link to ongoing career success and satisfaction. One study investigated the prevalence and effects of mentor relationships in the career development of 121 staff nurses. Their mentors were reportedly to have been particularly influential in their development, particularly in the early years of their practice. Seventy-one percent of the nurses rated having a mentor as very important in career development. Several helping relationships, in lieu of one exclusive mentor, were preferred (Johantgen, 1985). Another investigation of staff nurses reported that 95% of their mentors were both peers and nurse managers and that they perceived mentoring to be a large factor in their successful career development (Angelini, 1995). In a study of head nurses, it was found that a majority had mentors and that those who did were more likely to be mentors to others. A statistically significant relationship was present between age and head nurses who had mentors, that is, mentored head nurses were younger. In other words, those who had mentors attained a higher career level at an earlier age (Hyland-Hill, 1986). A survey of more than 500 clinical nurse specialists showed that those who had mentoring relationships indicated a significantly higher level of job satisfaction than those who did not have mentors (Caine, 1989a).

MENTORING THROUGHOUT A CAREER

A professional model of career development that is useful in understanding the central importance of mentor relationships throughout a career was developed by Dalton, Thompson, and Price (1977). This model describes four successive career stages—apprentice, colleague, mentor, and sponsor—and the primary relationships, central activities and tasks, and major issues and adjustments in each stage. Table 2.2 illustrates the key features of this career developmental model.

Clues to the mentoring activities of the professional nurse at various stages of the nursing career are available to us through a growing body of research and anecdotal reports. In an extensive literature

TABLE 2.2 Four Career Stages

Aspect	Stage 1	Stage 2	Stage 3	Stage 4
Primary Relationship	Apprentice Subordinate	Peer-Colleague	Mentor	Sponsor
Central activity or task	Helping Learning Following directions	Independent contributor	Training Influencing Interfacing	Shaping direction of the organization and profession
Major issues	Dependence	Independence	Assuming responsibility for others	Exercising power and influence

Source. Adapted from Dalton, Thompson, and Price (1977). Copyright 1977 by *Organizational Dynamics*. Adapted with permission.

review of the experience of mentorship, Swazey and Anderson (1996) note that the greatest portion of the literature has emerged from the nursing profession. Research and literature reviews on mentor-protégé relationships throughout the nursing career have been compiled by Jowers and Herr (1990), Vance and Olson (1991), and Olson and Vance (1998). A summary of 81 nursing research studies on mentorship conducted in the 15-year period from 1977–1992 provides data about the significant relationships and developmental tasks at various career points (Olson & Vance, 1993). Both the structure and process of mentorship are important parameters of these studies, including the presence of mentoring activity, who performs mentoring functions, and the types and outcomes of mentoring activities.

CAREER STAGE 1.

The first 2 years of a nursing career are often fraught with ambiguity and stress. The central task of this stage is to learn and to work with supervision, following directions and getting help from more experienced colleagues. Appropriately, the novice nurse should serve as an apprentice to competent mentors, learning the culture, professional judgment, and decision-making skills from observation and trial and correction. In this stage of exploration, mentors serve as intellectual guides and sociocultural role models, as suggested in the Super/Vance paradigm (see Table 2.1). Neophyte nurses gain the ability to use their intuition, knowledge, and experience in "putting the pieces together" with guidance and role modeling from willing mentors (Pyles & Stern, 1983). Benner's classic study *From Novice to Expert* (1984) describes the developmental stages through which a novice nurse must proceed to become a skillful, proficient practitioner: novice, advanced beginner, competent, proficient, expert. There is a compelling need for careful mentoring at each of these stages. One of the major issues in the first career stage is adjusting to the dependence inherent in the role of subordinate/neophyte practitioner. On the one hand, the new nurse has anticipated completing the rigorous course of study and, free of teachers' supervision, looks forward to being an independent practitioner. The new nurse, armed with a credential and license to practice, is compensated with a respectable entry-level salary and, therefore, is expected to perform quickly at a fairly high level, often autonomously. Indeed, the most helpful way of entering a professional career is frequently violated in hospitals and other acute care settings, where the majority of nurses begin their practice. The reality of traditional role expectations, an economic, bottom-line climate, and the complex demands of health care organizations frequently preclude adequate support for the new nurse. In spite of these barriers, finding caring mentors should be a major developmental task for every professional person entering an organization. Providing this opportunity is an equally important responsibility of the clinical and educational organizations, as well as advanced colleagues and peers.

Research investigations reveal the positive influence of mentorship during career entry. A study of 157 full-time, female nurses each of whom worked at least 1 year as a staff nurse in an acute care hospital revealed that a majority (73%) of the sample had at least two or more mentors who were older staff nurses or preceptors. Their mentors were acquired during the 1st year of employment, and the relationship lasted an average of 2 ½ years. There was a significant difference between the mean professionalism scores of mentored and nonmentored nurses, with mentored nurses achieving higher scores (Just, 1989). In a study of beginning nurses' diagnostic reasoning behaviors, a high level of beginner uncertainty and problems with independent diagnostic reasoning were found. The need for consistent consultation and carefully planned, novice nurse mentoring was demonstrated (Haffer, 1990). An investigation of neophyte nurses in critical care units suggested that whether they will achieve success depends a great deal on their adequate socialization into that world. Mentor relationships and experience were identified as the most important factors in the neophytes' development in making accurate patient assessments and nursing judgments (Pyles, 1981). An examination of a sample of 143 staff nurses revealed that 65% of them had one or several people help them advance in their nursing careers. The relationship with the support person most frequently began during the 1st year of work. An important finding is that almost a third of the respondents indicated that the support relationship began during elementary or secondary school or college. The study suggests that without a preceptor or mentor relationship, job dissatisfaction is more difficult to manage (Carey & Campbell, 1994).

The important entry issues into the profession include skill building, critical thinking, problem solving, decision making, prioritizing, developing self-confidence, and obtaining career guidance. Studies of the new nurse demonstrate that mentor relationships enhance skill building and strengthen self-confidence. Appropriately, the new nurse should function as a protégé under the tutelage of involved, caring, supportive, and experienced professionals. Novice nurses need affirmation in their new role and guidance during this tender socialization phase. Anecdotal evidence suggests that they frequently begin their careers in highly stressful, unsupportive, and demanding environments. There is reportedly an inadequate supply of mentors, the presence of "queen-beeism," and organizational climates that isolate, alienate, and foster passivity. In contrast to mentoring, there sometimes occurs "professional hazing," a phenomenon in which neophytes are made to prove themselves and their competency in an atmosphere of hostile challenge, lack of support, and difficult assignments. By contrast, when involved, caring mentors are available for beginning nurses, a foundation of work satisfaction and success, self-confidence, and professional commitment is established. Indeed, the benefits are accrued by not only the protégé, but by the mentors, the workplace, and the profession (Vance, 1989–90, 1992).

Mentor Remembered

(Anonymous, in Schorr, 1979. Reprinted with permission.)

Today I read your editorial in the November 1978 *American Journal of Nursing.* It was a revelation. It supplied a word I had been searching for to describe someone: "mentor."

When I entered a nursing program . . . , I had all the fears and doubts that any 29-year-old wife and mother develops when plunging into such an endeavor. Would I be able to compete with younger students? Could I develop good study habits? How would my children (then 4 and 6 years old) cope? How much encouragement would my busy husband be able to give? Did I have the guts to be a nurse? Would I faint at the sight of blood? Death? How would I confront pain? Insanity?

What I needed was a mentor. I needed someone to help me discover that the answers to those questions lay within me, that the potential for coping was there.

I remember her on the first day of classes, smiling, barely audible. She was rather shy in front of us. I admired her smart clothes and her stylish hair-do. (Many weeks later I discovered she wore a wig. Radiation treatments for cancer had claimed her own hair.) She spoke in a lilting accent and had a dry, quiet wit.

We became friends, though always retaining the respectful spaces of the teacher-student relationship. Even now, I have difficulty using her first name.

She encouraged, cajoled, teased, scolded, and prayed all of her students through school. Mostly, though, she taught by example. One semester, she left us to have serious surgery. We worried, but she came back smiling, telling us how one "really does become disoriented in ICU," and demonstrating new techniques she'd been a guinea pig for.

Another time we saw her torn by indecision. She told us quietly that her oncologist had recommended a prophylactic course of chemotherapy to supplement radiation. She frowned a few times during those weeks of indecision. Finally she told the doctors, "No." She taught all of us the meaning of nursing, but she taught me especially well because she instinctively knew two things about me, first, that I was her kindred spirit, and second, that I was bound to be a nurse.

Signing R.N. after my name is no longer as thrilling as it was when I first received my license. She and I no longer see each other frequently. Yet every time I walk into a patient's room, I think I imagine her bending over the patient's bed, knowing by some indefinable perception that the patient needs to be repositioned.

I can almost see, with her eyes, every detail. The I.V.—what's in it? Is it running at the correct rate? Is the site normal in appearance? Is there other equipment that needs to be tended to? What is the patient's state of mind? Does he need to be touched or held at arm's length? Will a smile or a joke help, or is some serious listening needed?

Then there are the days when I wake and say, "I can't make it today. I'm too tired," or "I don't feel well." But then I visualize her working in spite of her pain and weakness, and I get on with my day.

It seems to me that she was there the first time I did everything: made a bed ("You'll never bounce a quarter off that"); wrote a care plan; gave an IM to an orange; inserted a catheter (into the vagina!); made 100% on a test; made 70% on a test; saw my first operation (without fainting); heard that one of my patients had died; found out that I had a painful, chronic disease; cried because I couldn't ease a patient's pain; cried because I could; laughed when there seemed to be absolutely nothing else to do.

The "firsts" are fewer now, but her spirit still prevails. I would have become a nurse without her, but never would I have sought the level of professionalism, the degree of compassion, the depth of humor, the height of empathy that are set as guideposts for me by the conduct of my mentor.

CAREER STAGE 2.

From approximately 3 to 10 years in the field, the nurse must become an increasingly competent and highly skilled professional who can work independently and make a significant contribution to the organization and the profession. Specialization occurs through advanced study and work training. The nurse becomes increasingly self-confident and visible in the organization. This is the colleague stage, and peer mentoring is a common phenomenon. At the same time, expert professionals also are serving as mentors through the various transitions occurring at this stage: deciding on a specialty area, engaging in graduate study, achieving specialty certification, assuming a different professional role, and juggling professional and family life. Growing independence occurs, with increased confidence in judgment and in skills, along with a deepening professional and career commitment. In this stage, clinicians, graduate students, managers, nurse educators, and researchers seek mentoring support from both peers and advanced-level nurses. The mentor's gifts are encouragement, guidance, inspiration, and belief in

the nurse's growing competence. This career point is consistent with the
Super/Vance stage of expansion (Table 2.1), in which the mentor serves
as a visionary-idealist and a promoter-coach. Here the nurse is assisted
with role expansion and balancing; advanced education; facilitation of
clinical, managerial, teaching, and research skill development; career
promotion; and networking opportunities.

A predominant difference between traditional mentoring and
peer-collegial mentoring has been found through empirical investigation and nurses' stories about mentoring. Nurses engage in traditional expert-to-novice mentoring, but, in addition, many of them
attest to the central importance of peer-collegial mentoring throughout their personal and career development. At each developmental
stage, many nurses turn to trusted peer-colleagues for support and
friendship. These peers often become lifelong, long-distance friends.
Nurses' professional lives consist of many transition points, and the
support and guidance of peers become central in achieving a successful and happy resolution at these junctures. The career and personal
transition points reported by nurses include applying for scholar-
ships, entering graduate school, completing academic degrees, changing or losing a job, deciding on or changing a specialty area, being
promoted, seeking tenure, getting married, becoming a parent, moving, confronting a family death, and breaking into research and publishing arenas. The intermix of professional and personal developmental
challenges for nurses and women seems to call for the type of mentoring assistance that peers can provide. Faced with the complexities
and challenges of contemporary life, we suggest that nurses and nursing students cultivate both traditional (expert) mentors and nontraditional (peer) mentors.

Research studies provide data about this career stage and nurses'
mentor connections. In an investigation of nurse managers in hospitals, those who had mentors reported greater role clarity and higher
satisfaction with career opportunities than those not having mentors
(Dunsmore, 1987). Of 100 nurse managers in another study, 79%
reported having mentors, with the most significant mentoring relationships occurring in superior-to-subordinate relationships and peer
relationships. These managers reported that their careers were affected
significantly by mentors during the early years of their careers (Boyle
& James, 1990). Sixty-three nurse practitioners identified counseling,
educating, sponsoring, and commitment to both the protégé and the
profession as important components of their mentoring relationships.
It was suggested that a mentoring program, as part of the educational

curriculum for nurse practitioners, is important for role socialization (Freeman, 1989). Faculty protégé-mentor relationships were explored with more than 250 faculty members in baccalaureate nursing programs. Mentors were found to be very important in helping novice faculty members get into the system, become socialized to the sociopolitical climate, and take on responsibilities with the mentor. Mentoring did not, however, increase faculty involvement in publishing, research, professional organizations, university committees, and community service (Macey, 1985). Nurse educator mentors and protégés (N = 153) reported that participation in a mentor relationship enhanced their career satisfaction (Olson, 1984). Another study examined the extent to which mentor relationships between senior and junior faculty (N = 183) influenced the research productivity of the junior faculty. It was found that a collaborative model of mentorship and coparticipation of mentors with protégés promoted research productivity of both mentor and protégé (Williams, 1986; Williams & Blackburn, 1988). Two large studies of nurse faculty revealed significant mentoring activity and the important role that the organization can play in the promotion of effective mentoring experiences (Tagg, 1986; Vogt, 1985). Research studies of the nurse in expanding roles suggest that mentor relationships enhance career commitment and work and personal satisfaction. These helping relationships assist in role socialization and role clarity as specialization and advancement occur. It is evident that those who have mentoring assistance achieve at higher levels because progress is easier and faster. Nurses also report a variety of support influences, including traditional mentors and peer-colleagues, these influences being especially valuable at transition points. Peer-collegial support is highlighted as particularly valuable. Indeed, the line between peer mentor and friend is often evanescent. Friends and mentors guide and learn from each other, especially in unexplored terrain (Bateson, 1990). Organizational climate and leadership also play an important role in promoting effective mentor experiences—both traditional and peer collegial. There are reciprocal benefits for the mentor and the protégé, as well as for the organization and the profession.

CAREER STAGE 3.

Nurses in this stage, generally having been in the profession between 10 and 20 years, assume increased responsibility for influencing, guiding, directing, and developing others. This is the mentor stage. Professionals in this stage assume several roles, including mentor,

manager and administrator and idea person. They exhibit broadened
capabilities and interests, both within and outside their organizations.
Their work is complex, requiring a high degree of interpersonal skill
level, with high rewards and high satisfaction. Academic and service
administrators, advanced practice nurses, and researchers are mentoring others in earlier career stages and their peers at the same time
they are continuing to receive mentoring support from colleagues and
those in more advanced positions. As mentors, these leaders derive
deep satisfaction from watching their protégés develop leadership
abilities. This is the time for recognizing and preparing promising
members of the profession for advancement and leadership succession. Studies of advanced-level nurses demonstrate that there is a
prevalence of mentoring activity among them. Those who have been
mentored will mentor others, thus creating a generational effect. A
variety of mentor connections is created as these leaders assume
responsibility for others and at the same time receive support. These
connections are essential for the development of leadership advancement and succession. The commitment of the leadership and the organization to mentorship is a critical factor in the promotion of effective
mentor connections.

    In one study, nursing leaders—from head nurses to top-level
administrators—in hospital settings were investigated in relation to
their work satisfaction. A replication of that study also was performed.
Major findings from both studies revealed that those who have mentors are likely to be mentors; satisfaction with work, superiors, and
coworkers was higher in those who have mentors; and satisfaction
with work was higher in those who were mentors to others. Mentors
were nursing administrators and supervisors, nurse educators, and
peer-colleagues (Giese, 1986; Larson, 1980, 1986). A survey of 427 academic administrators provides clues about mentoring and career
development in the profession. Significant differences between mentored and nonmentored subjects were found in relation to the number
of publications, grant funding successes, and level of career development scores. Mentored subjects were younger, and a greater number
of them held doctorates than did the nonmentored subjects. The
researchers speculated on the mentors' influence on these administrators in pursuing higher degrees, with the concomitant outcomes inherent in becoming better educated and better prepared, that is,
publishing more, receiving grants, and becoming more fully developed in their careers (Rawl, 1989; Rawl & Peterson, 1992). Two hundred seventy-four female nursing service executives in medical center

hospitals were surveyed for information on the existence and nature of their mentoring relationships. Seventy-one percent stated that they had a mentor, who was usually older than they, held a higher organizational position, with the relationship lasting 1 to 5 years. The most reported beneficial mentor behavior was showing confidence in the protégé. The greater the emotional commitment to the protégé, the greater the effect on career development (Holloran, 1989).

Mentoring for Succession

by Margery Adams and Edward Beard, Jr.

At Catawba Memorial Hospital in Hickory, North Carolina, a mentoring relationship prepared a nurse for succession to the office of Vice President of Patient Services. Margery Adams, the Vice President of Patient Services at the time, was preparing to retire within 5 years. After 20 years of developing a professional nursing practice at the hospital, Margery's goal was to preserve the progress that had been made in caring for patients. Edward Beard, Jr., a nursing administration student at the University of North Carolina at Greensboro, was a graduate intern at the hospital who was being preceptored by Margery. This became a successful outcome-oriented mentoring relationship for succession.

EB: I launched into the role of administrative intern with a vengeance. I found that Margery was willing to involve me in all aspects of her role, and I had no reservation about commenting on or asking anything. There was no thought of being put down or of "positional" power. I freely observed and inquired about everything she did. She patiently responded to my inquisitions, as I wanted to know "why" about everything.

MA: From the beginning, I found Eddie to be an eager learner, academically knowledgeable, and capable of asking many questions. Early in the internship he demonstrated he could apply what he learned. He began to assist in problem solving, to comment on how situations should be resolved, and to argue for his opinion. He became an asset as he researched projects, responded to hospital personnel, wrote reports, and made presentations.

EB: Near the end of my mentored preceptorship, Margery began questioning me about my plans for the future. Would I be willing to relocate? She insisted that I describe what type of position I really wanted—and so I told her the truth—"yours." I did not know at the time that she was exploring my interest in taking a position with her.

MA: I recognized a special aptitude and talent in Eddie that I wanted for our hospital. He did all the right things—he was well mannered, poised, willing and helpful, even as a student. He had become involved in a project that continued beyond his internship and requested permission to return on his own time to see the conclusion. I decided to create a position for Eddie and to mentor him into my position. During part of our negotiations, he said that he would be ready to take my place in about a year. I knew then I had made no mistake; this young man was not "finished" yet. I was very interested in helping him reach his goal and supporting his abilities to move our nursing service into shared governance, case management, and the information age.

EB: I approached work with an attitude of overconfidence, thinking I knew it all. In this early phase, Margery provided carefully selected assignments. They seemed so carefully selected that at times I was bored. I wanted to do more. But the minute I became an employee, "positional" power became an issue. We had discussed the fact that achieving acceptance from others would take time. I knew that, but was impatient and wanted to become quickly involved in every aspect of the nurse executive role. In retrospect, easing me in has proven advantageous in developing strong, long-term relationships with hospital personnel. I credit Margery with the insight that an initial "wrong" impression, no matter how innocent, is almost impossible to overcome.

MA: Early on, my challenge was to get Eddie accepted as an employee. His status as a student had been well received. I realized the risk of being in a new position and was very cautious to design and assign successful projects and positive encounters. Almost a year into his employment, we discussed his goal of reaching the chief nurse executive role in 1 year. By then, reality had hit, and his expectations were adjusted. We were able to plan and implement a shared governance structure, improve our data management, and concentrate on needed change and progress.

EB: After I settled into the job for a period of time, the phase of introducing me to the nurse executive community began.

With Margery's years of experience and respect among colleagues, getting me to the right place to meet the right people was easy for her. It was not easy for me. I was confronted with the task of putting names with faces and presenting myself in a manner not to embarrass her. To become "known," I was assigned formal presentations, with no escape, and I suffered from stage fright.

MA: I refused to allow Eddie to surrender to fears and old habits. "I can't remember names" was not acceptable. I explained that to remember was required, and now he remembers everyone. Many times I have wished someone had helped me with public speaking. Following two important failures at public speaking with only a few minor successes, I declared I would do no more public speaking. I was determined not to have this happen to him. Together we wrote interesting, creative presentations, rehearsed them, and success came. He is well on the way to being a fine public speaker.

EB: As time passed, Margery began to give me more and more freedom to introduce new ideas and programs. Creating and expanding programs excited me. This new freedom allowed me the opportunity to explore and further develop my nursing values. I gained experience in personnel matters, group process, hospitalwide projects and, at last, in every aspect of the nurse executive role. This is the time I developed management wisdom and skill. My natural tendency was toward feeling rather than thinking. I experienced the value of questioning and listening before deciding. I learned that timing is everything; that if I asked a question I had to deal with its answer; that "seeking forgiveness beats asking permission"; and that it is always acceptable to "eat an elephant one bite at a time."

MA: The process of taking over the reins took place during the last 18 months of our 5-year mentored relationship. As Eddie assumed more and more responsibility, I positioned myself on the sideline to observe and critique. In most instances, we talked over approaches and strategies in advance, and my role became a presence for support—the silent partner. I accepted him as a true and worthy colleague.

MA and EB: During our 5-year mentor-protégé relationship, our intent was to role model professionalism, mutual respect, and an openness to discuss and debate issues. Today we believe we have come full circle, as one of us leaves a long-held position and one of us assumes full responsibility for it. We believe we have had the best of everything these last 5 years. Margery believes in storytelling and has shared many stories, and Eddie has been a willing listener. Margery believes that knowledge and skills shared with others are the ones that will remain forever. The sense of history gained in hearing stories and the shaping of thought processes and defining of values have made Eddie secure and confident. Eddie is ready to go it alone. We have learned that for our values to be renewed, we must be willing to share them with others. To do this takes willingness, trust, and time. Commitment to sharing through mentorship will ensure that our values will be given away over and over again. Eddie will now seek opportunities to carry on another generation of mentoring as taught by Margery, his mentor.

CAREER STAGE 4.

Nurses in this stage exert a wide sphere of influence, shaping the direction of the organizations in which they work, as well as external organizations and the profession. They exercise influence by negotiating and interfacing with key aspects of the environment, developing new ideas, markets, or services, and directing the resources of the organization toward specific goals (Dalton et al., 1977). Nurse-influentials can be found in various roles; exercising power and influence are part of their daily lives. Forming extensive networks and alliances as well as formulating policy are part of their armamentarium. They communicate through extensive speaking and writing activities. Multiple mentors have frequently assisted these leaders in their career development; and they in turn serve as mentor-sponsors to individuals, professional groups, and organizations. Their sponsorship prepares others to assume leadership for new roles or for succession. Through this sponsorship, they have the opportunity to shape and to transform organizations and the profession for the future. Indeed, mentorship on behalf of developing strong visionary leadership for the future is an obligation of a true leader. Studies reveal that influential leaders recognize the significant assistance that they received from their mentors. Their mentor connections have supported their leadership development and career advancement and frequently lead to friendship and collegial partnerships. Leaders understand the central importance of active mentorship and sponsorship of others, of lending their guidance and support. Through sharing their experiences and wisdom, leaders further evolve their own strength and extend their influence throughout the profession. They therefore influence the future direction of the profession and of organizations through extensive collegial mentor connections. In describing long-distance leaders or "success sustainers" who keep their pursuit of excellence in balance with their inner well-being, O'Neil (1993) states that welcoming opportunities to teach and serve as a mentor to others is one of their characteristics. They are promoters of human growth and professional development. Mentor-leaders' stock-in-trade is the future, and they invest wisely in human potential and power.

Nationally recognized nurse-influentials (N = 71) were surveyed regarding their sources and activities of influence. Eighty-three percent reported having mentors, while 93% reported being mentors to many protégés. Multiple mentors provided different types of assistance at various points in their careers. Types of help received by their mentors included: (a) career advice, guidance, and promotion; (b) professional role modeling; (c) intellectual and scholarly stimulation; (d) inspiration and idealism; (e) teaching and advising; and (f) emotional support (Vance, 1977). A decade later, a replication study compared these influentials with a later group and found a strong resemblance to the earlier group in relation to their mentor activity. Career advice, guidance, and promotion were the predominant mentoring activities (Kinsey, 1985, 1986). In another study, 57% of more than 500 doctorally prepared nurses reported having at least one mentor. Comparisons between mentored and nonmentored subjects indicated that those with mentors followed a definitive career plan more frequently, were more satisfied with their career progress, and had a greater sense of accomplishment. Satisfaction with their mentoring relationships was high—99.2% (Spengler, 1982). Nursing leaders of national and state organizations described the presence of extensive mentorship experiences by intensity, definition, role, and professional phase. The definition of "mentorship" for national leaders was "professional friendship," and for state leaders, it was "pragmatic experience" (Lee, 1988). Sixty-four percent of a sample of 44 Fellows of the American Academy of Nursing reported having mentor relationships that were a significant factor in their career development. These relationships became increasingly collegial partnerships or friendships. These leaders were actively mentoring other nurses (Slagle, 1986). Nursing administrators from one large hospital were studied through an ethnographic approach (participant observation and in-depth interviews), with the cultural theme of survival emerging as most significant. It was emphasized that most nurse administrators learn successful survival strategies and informal rules by trial and error, and that hospitals could provide greater assistance and support by developing mentorship programs based on relationships between experienced and new administrators (Garner, 1995). A profile of 324 influential, academic nurse administrators was developed by Short (1994, 1997b). Mentoring played a key role in their development as well as networking, role models, and advanced education. Over 70% reported the presence of mentoring, and 89% were serving as mentors to others. It was found that at the dean's level, however, opportunities for obtaining a mentor seemed to diminish.

According to Short, there was a variety of reasons for not having a mentor. Some of the administrators indicated a problem with the confidence levels of their associates and potential mentors. One person stated that "my boss has less education and experience than I do and is defensive;" another said that "my experience made me be perceived as a threat." Others discussed the lack of opportunity and claimed that the "environment . . . did not foster" mentoring relationships or that "no one ever offered" to be a mentor. A few commented on their difficulty in requesting help from anyone. Several of them indicated that they made use of other types of career supports, such as role models and networking. One dean said that she had "utilized the knowledge and skills of a variety of individuals," and another said that "I learned from observing and interacting with many of my professors and professional colleagues." Many of the deans had supportive collegial relationships, albeit not fitting the traditional mentoring concept.

THE MENTOR CONNECTION, NETWORKS, AND ROLE MODELS

The mentor connection is composed not only of mentor-sponsors and protégés, but also of role models and networks. The mentor connection implies a web of inclusion and connection (Gilligan, 1993; Helgesen, 1990). Mentoring assumes caring and connecting with one another.

These mentor connections of caring, in which mentors and protégés sustain and empower each other, create powerful networks for promoting growth and change within the profession and within the health care system and the larger society. These connections of caring are sources of power and influence for both mentor/leaders and protégé/rising stars. We believe that a high-order value for nursing, a predominantly female profession, is one of caring and thereby inclusion. The strategy of the web emphasizes strengthening interrelationships, "working to tighten them, building up strength, knitting loose ends into the fabric; it is a strategy that honors the feminine principles of inclusion and connection" (Helgesen, p. 58).

Mentor relationships naturally lead to networks and alliances in which the affiliative spirit of sharing and cooperation is present. These networks and alliances can lead to important collaborative endeavors among mentor-protégé dyads as well as in larger circles. In providing leadership and service to society, knowledge is essential, but people working together on behalf of shared values and shared experiences is equally essential. Mentor connections and networks are a requisite ingredient in this endeavor. Felton (1978) postulated that the paucity of women in positions of leadership, authority, and power in society stems from their lack of mentors and sponsors who can be instrumental in preparation and introduction to established networks that promote career progress and success.

Mentors serve as living role models. Nurse-influentials claimed that an essential component of the assistance provided by their mentors was professional role modeling, serving as exemplars of excellence to be imitated. They reported that their mentors were "role models for change and risk-taking and for political and diplomatic action"; "for what professional nursing should be"; and "teacher-models for scholarship, research, administration and delegation." In the Super/Vance paradigm (Table 2.1, p. 14), the sociocultural role model figures predominantly in the developmental stage of professional and personal exploration. The mentor-role model introduces and socializes the protégé to the profession—its values, customs, and members. Female mentors can serve as intensified role models for professional women in that they can model the blending of the unique female personal role and the professional work role. Female mentors can influence the transformation of these roles. Identification with the same-gender mentor-role model is a powerful mechanism for exploring societal and personal meaning, values, and experiences and ways to integrate these into a full and balanced life.

Reflections on Mentoring and Networks

by Geraldene Felton

To be educated assures a measure of freedom. I have lived my entire life to be as free as possible. Education has meant not only being literate and having a skill; it also has meant becoming increasingly competent in the science and technology necessary to be an expert in my discipline. It has involved a lifetime of learning and giving service. It has included involvement in a continuum of mentoring relationships by persons who have generously served as patrons, protectors, benefactors, sponsors, advocates, and advisers. My survival and career advancement were made possible by those who mentored me. Specifically, they:

- served as role models;
- provided career advice, suggestions, and guidance;
- gave recognition and encouragement;
- offered honest criticism and informal feedback;
- helped me form and maintain collaborative relationships; and
- guided me in becoming politically savvy.

Three individual mentors greatly influenced my career. They were a nursing instructor, the dean of a medical school who was a non-MD physiologist, and a vice president for academic affairs. The last two were instrumental during my transition into new positions. To speak of mentors is also to speak of networks. Networking is the deliberate process of reaching out to others and developing and using contacts for information, counsel, ideas, sponsorship, and moral support. It involves asking for mentoring when you need it and giving mentoring when others need it. Networking informs others of one's talents and abilities, and the nature of one's contributions. It also is an effective means of quickly mobilizing people to achieve desirable outcomes. Networks have provided access to information that I needed in the university setting, such as cues about the "shadow" organization, unwritten rules, necessary knowledge sets, and budgeting skills. This information is vital to survival and advancement, as is the sharing of information and strategies with colleagues who provide a sounding board, advice, and feedback on ideas and behavior. Such help has influenced me to take informed risks or has just made me feel more comfortable. It also has helped me believe in myself and my membership in a disciplined community. People are in networks because of the positions they hold, their interests, abilities, expertise, and connections. What this means is that network support is based on performance. Translated, this means one must be good at one's job and be able to communicate this to others. No amount of active networking can overcome incompetence or indifference, because no one in a network can afford to put her or his influence and credibility on the line for someone who clearly does not deserve it. Nor have I found it necessary to like everyone in my network. However, cordiality is necessary, as is mutual respect, having something to offer, and willingness to invest time and resources to participate in supportive exchanges and problem solving.

A passion for networking and serving as a mentor to younger faculty, academic colleagues, and graduate students means that tailoring environments has been part of my life—a formidable mental and physical challenge. My passion is based on the belief that if doctoral students and young faculty do not become protégés of productive established academicians, do not have resources to carry out their research and scholarly work, do not have access to collegial networks where useful advice, advocacy, and patronage are dispersed—they begin their careers with an initial disadvantage and may find that the disadvantage grows with time. We are at an age in nursing when there is a great need to increase both informal and formal mentor systems for faculty and clinical nurses holding junior ranks. In some institutions the values acquired during earlier phases of nursing's development have resulted in senior faculty and senior clinicians becoming so entrepreneurial that they have forgotten their professional responsibility to reach out with a helping hand to give advice to younger colleagues who may be struggling with their development. Maybe "forgotten" is the wrong word. Perhaps "too busy with their own preoccupations" is more accurate. What differentiates the mentor from the entrepreneur may be related to the individual's development as a person. A major difference is that mentors transcend their own interests, self-promotion and recognition needs, and share their talents with others. Leaders can foster mentoring behaviors. Moreover, giving recognition to senior colleagues who serve as mentors is exceedingly important, not only because it is well deserved but because it also assists them to have the psychological strength to continue these important behaviors.

3

Women Mentoring Women: Nurse to Nurse

That women must redefine the mentoring relationship in their own terms to meet their unique needs is a bold, new idea. Rather than struggle to make the male model fit, women must create a new model if they are to fulfill their own potential (Jeruchim & Shapiro, 1992).

Mentorship has not been considered part of the experience of most women until recently. The phenomenon of women mentoring women was not an area of serious study or investigation in American society until the late 1970s. Although historically, women in work, home, community, social, and religious settings have supported and assisted each other through family and friendship connections, the label of "mentoring" was never placed on these relationships. It was not until women in large numbers entered professional, academic, and corporate settings that they became acquainted with the "old boys' network" and male mentor relationships. Clearly, mentor connections and networks were integral to the developmental experience of successful career-oriented men. Indeed, it was suggested that "everyone who makes it has a mentor" and that mentors are essential to advancing in the workplace (Collins & Scott, 1978; Roche, 1979). Women began to recognize that without these mentor connections they were "out of the loop" and seriously hampered in their professional development. Access to vital information, networks, and political know-how and support was severely limited without mentor networks.

Although studies about women and their mentors are still relatively rare, those that have been conducted lend credence to the enormous importance of the presence of mentors for women's career development and success. Two decades ago the "mentor connection" was depicted as the secret link in the successful woman's life (Sheehy, 1976). It was found that almost without exception, women who had gained recognition in their careers were at some point nurtured by mentors. The career development of women executives was studied by Hennig (1970), who reported that their career success would not have been possible without the relationship they had established with their bosses—a type of patron-protégé relationship. A "protégé" was described as someone whose welfare, training, or career is promoted by an influential person or patron (Hennig & Jardim, 1977). In a study of a large corporation, Kanter and Stein (1979) found that women who were not successful in the company were without a support system of mentors. More than 400 professional women were surveyed by Collins (1983), who found that although 75% of them had male mentors, they were not sophisticated in seeking mentors. Over half of the women surveyed reported that they "fell into" the relationship rather than fully comprehending its value.

In spite of the importance of mentors for career success, many women have not experienced this type of support. They were frequently presumed to lack commitment and drive, and, therefore, were not seen as worthy or serious protégés. Other reasons given for women not having mentors include the lack of female role models, women's failure to mentor other women, the potential sexual aspects of male-female mentor relationships, and the lack of serious attention given to female talent (Bolton, 1980). One writer, lamenting the difficulty for a woman to obtain a mentor, claimed it is probably more important for her to have a mentor than it is for a man to rise or gain notice in a field because of the continuing discrimination against women in the workplace (Epstein, 1970).

A conference that explored the subject of women and success concluded that women rarely find support among their female peers even though the development of a career woman's confidence and self-esteem depends upon this support (Kundsin, 1974). In a 15-year biographical study of 45 female academics, corporate executives, and homemakers that commenced in the early 1980s, Levinson (1996) found that only one third of the professional women had mentors. Throughout their careers, they continued to be hampered in developing full professional achievement by the lack of mentoring assistance.

In addition to the lack of readily accessible mentors, women's career development often has been complicated by late career selection and specialization, delayed credentialing, frequent career interruptions, and fewer advancement opportunities (Noe, 1988a, 1988b; Shapiro, Haseltine, & Rowe, 1978). Female professionals, therefore, bring a unique set of challenges to their careers: juggling the multiple roles of a private (e.g., motherhood) and public life, traditional sex-role conditioning, lack of career planning, diminished access to power structures, devaluation of traditional women's work, and diminished self-esteem. A 7-year study of 676 women holding master's degrees in business administration demonstrated that even at the present time women are not being groomed, promoted, or paid at the same level as their male counterparts, despite having proved themselves in the workplace (Schneer & Retiman, 1995). Many of these women reported that they had to work harder than male colleagues to attain leadership positions.

As the millennium approaches, women are increasingly finding their way in large numbers in the workplace and in academia. Women now represent about half of the American workforce. Ninety-seven percent of employed nurses are women. Women also are discovering their "voices." They are becoming more visible in leadership positions. They are acting on behalf of their values and dreams. Professional women, including nurses, now seem more willing to transform rather than adopt willy-nilly the male norms of work and social issues (Campbell-Heider, 1986). Obstacles still exist, however, for the full and equitable integration, development, and recognition of professional women in the workplace. These obstacles are frequently a result of powerful social norms and a welter of old assumptions about women's and men's natures (Aisenberg & Harrington, 1988). Studies of women's career development suggest that one of the major barriers to their participation in a fully developed career as well as negatively influenced opportunities for career advancement is the scarcity of role models, mentor connections, and networks.

In the last 2 decades, many questions about mentorship for women have been raised in the business, educational, nursing, and other professional fields. What is the nature of mentoring? To what extent is it available for female professionals? Who best serve as mentors to women? How does mentoring assist in career development and success? What are the barriers to forming mentor connections? Early investigations of the mentorship phenomenon have provided useful information. We can now state with greater precision what mentoring is, including key characteristics, benefits, and barriers. Studies show, for example, that many career women have mentor relationships, although these are still scarce and not always easy to develop and to sustain. We also know with certainty that mentors are important for personal and professional growth. Mentorship is increasingly documented as integral to leadership development (Altieri & Elgin, 1994; McCloskey & Molen, 1987). Clearly, female professionals have a great need and desire for mentors.

The nursing profession did not address the mentor concept in its literature and research until the late 1970s. The first study to investigate mentor relationships occurring among nursing leaders in the United States was conducted by Vance (1977). This study of 71 nationally identified nurse-influentials provided an early illustration of the nature of the mentoring process for successful female professionals. These leaders described in detail the relationships with their mentors and protégés. It is important to note that every one of them reported that she had received mentoring help from a variety of support relationships with peer colleagues, work supervisors, teachers, other professionals, friends, and relatives, in addition to "traditional" mentors. Their mentor relationships supported the notion of mentoring occurring on a continuum of mentor-sponsor-guide-peer pal, as reported by Shapiro et al. (1978). The nurse-influentials chronicled the significant influences that their mentors played at various career points. Different influences were important at different points in their careers. The emphasis on the type of help changed from period to period or from one transition to the next. The importance of finding a mentor who can help with career growth in one's area of interest was reported in a survey of influential academic nurse administrators (Short, 1994, 1997a, 1997b). The value of having a series of mentors also was highlighted by these leaders. These studies of nurse-influentials highlight the value of possessing various resources for goal achievement, such as communication skills and advanced education, and concomitant mentor relationships to facilitate the development and actualization of these resources.

Because the nursing profession is composed primarily of women (97%), empirical studies and stories about mentoring in nursing provide important clues to an evolving female model of mentorship and insights into women's personal and professional development. The process of women's mentor relationships merits scrutiny, including the supports and barriers, positive and negative aspects, and the reciprocal nature and phases of these relationships. For example, female nurse administrators have been studied for clarification of the mentoring process that occurs with high-level leaders. The data illustrate active involvement in mentoring activity, as both mentor and protégé, in relationships that often exceed 25 years. Some negative aspects have been reported in a few studies, usually related to competition and control. The majority of mentored and nonmentored leaders strongly advocate mentor connections for career development, advancement, and satisfaction.

These issues are illustrated in the following research findings of female nursing leaders. The major factors influencing the career success of 236 doctorally prepared women in nursing were identified as personal characteristics, educational preparation, and significant others (Zimmerman, 1983). Their most influential mentors were teachers, peers, and work supervisors. Three hundred female academic nurse administrators were surveyed, with 93% reporting one or more career mentors. They reported that similar personalities were not critical to their mentor relationships and that their relationships remained friendly in spite of differences (White, 1986, 1988). The mentoring experiences and career satisfaction of 130 Black female administrators revealed that 80% had mentors and those who had multifaceted types of professional support were more satisfied with their careers than those lacking this support (Malone, 1981). A sample of 19 female chief nurse executives identified positive role models who had influenced their professional development. The majority of their role models also were their mentors. Each of these leaders believed that she had a commitment to mentor her subordinates in a cycle of mentorship (Redmond, 1995). Ten female administrators of baccalaureate nursing programs who had mentors participated in a greater number of career development activities, completed doctorates earlier, and moved into administrative positions sooner than nonmentored subjects (Bahr, 1985). Significant others were identified by 372 deans of nursing as one of the major influences in their life-career pathway. Many persons, especially women, played quasi-mentoring roles throughout these deans' development, providing role modeling and sponsorship (Redmond, 1991).

Because the academy continues to be male dominated, various forms of support and development for female faculty and students are necessary for full integration and development. For example, it has been estimated that only about 15% of academics on tenure tracks are women (Levinson, 1996). The concern for women and educational equity is contained in the Platform for Action from the United Nations

Fourth World Conference on Women held in Beijing in 1995 and adopted by 189 world governments, including the United States. Strengthening opportunities and access for girls and women throughout their lives to education, career development, support, and teaching is part of the educational agenda (United Nations, Department of Public Information, 1996). Speaking of her success in improving the educational retention rates of minority women, a nurse educator stated that minority mentors are dramatically needed at all levels of education. "Mentoring assists the student to unlock the bars of internal or external prejudice when it exists . . . and encourages the minority woman to develop behaviors which help her view her educational setting realistically" (Nelson, 1995, p. 365). Another author suggested that mentoring holds great potential for transforming the academy. By strengthening the values of collaboration, connectedness, and caring, which are essential to quality mentoring, an academic institution can be transformed into one that is truly a "community" of scholars (Johnsrud, 1991).

Studies of female nursing faculty demonstrate the strong presence of mentors and underscore the critical importance of these mentors for understanding the norms and values of the academy, for career growth, and for continued success in the academic role. More than 300 doctorally prepared female nursing school faculty were surveyed to establish the relationship between mentoring for the academic role and scholarly productivity. The length, timing, and nature of the mentoring, including the types of support provided by the mentor, were found to influence scholarly productivity. Mentorships that enhanced scholarly productivity occurred when protégés sensed an intense relationship, friendship, and philosophical similarity with their mentors (Butler, 1989). Kremgold-Barrett's 1986 study, "Women Mentoring Women in an Academic Nursing Facility," suggested that collegiality, affirmation, role modeling, and active mentoring are necessary for successful assimilation into the academy and for achieving tenure. A sense of mastery and competence also is important in attracting an appropriate support system. A survey of mentor relationships among 477 female nurse academicians concluded that the mentor is a positive, pivotal figure in their academic lives, especially as a role model and master teacher and in inspiring self-confidence. The mentor, however, did not strongly influence research and scholarly endeavors, with a lack of collaboration in these areas between mentor and protégé (Taylor, 1992). A sample of female nursing faculty reported that their experiences as protégés contributed to the socialization of academic values, development of professional skills, and the enhancement of professional opportunities. All agreed that having a mentor made a difference in their career progress. The mentor connection most frequently began as a faculty-student relationship, changed over time (becoming more collegial or more like a friendship), and lasted from 4 to 33 years (Powell, 1990).

Out of her concern for strengthening the developmental relationships among women and nurses, Caroline Wright developed and led Mentor Workshops throughout Australia in the late 1980s.

My Story about Women's and Nurses' Mentor Relationships

by Caroline M. Wright

The Mentor Workshops included nursing academics, students, and clinical practitioners. I found that what is common to all of these women is that they remain humane and nurturing in their developmental relationships with other women despite many structural work barriers. During these workshops, it became clear that mentoring offers an alternative model of nurture and support for nurses (who are primarily women) that is different from and transcends the traditional models of supervision promulgated by a male-driven bureaucratic paradigm. The differences are illustrated below:

Mentorship (Feminine)	Supervision (Masculine)
Affiliative	Nonaffiliative
Mutual Learning	Expert/Neophyte
Supportive	Directive
Egalitarian	Authoritarian
Process Oriented	Task Oriented
Intuitive, Responsive	Planned, Static
Feelings	Analysis
Cooperative	Structured
Chosen Relationship	Compelled Relationship

It is my contention that nurses develop nurturing professional values over time as they practice their profession. These nurturing professional values extend not only to clients but to colleagues as well. It is these nurturing professional values that need to be acknowledged and strengthened further if we want to increase the numbers and types of mentor relationships in nursing. The "nurse-story" that I share with nursing colleagues who are female is that I believe we can and do relate to each other in more collegial, cooperative, and developmental ways than many men in business and careers. Although we work in patriarchal and authoritarian, bureaucratic organizations that usually do not recognize, value, or reward this form of interaction and support, it is imperative that we develop different structures that will facilitate our mentoring of each other. The establishment of these developmental mentor relationships with each other becomes a reward in itself. These relationships are a gift to each other. It is my belief that nurses are wise and mature enough to plan together to strengthen our mentor connections. A new social order awaits our calling if we work together to reform the structure of the current system. If the rules are inappropriate for the majority of health care workers, then let's change them.

In summary, studies of mentoring relationships among female nurses illustrate several features:

- mentoring is a common occurrence;
- their mentors are usually female;
- support comes from a variety of mentors: teachers, peer-colleagues, and work superiors;
- the mentor relationship occurs through various career stages and transitions, is long term, and characterized by growing collegiality and/or friendship;
- those who have been mentored mentor others;
- the major components of mentor relationships are career development and enhancement activities, role modeling, professional socialization, affirmation, recognition of potential, and inspiration; and
- competence and commitment are important in attracting mentoring support.

TWO WORLD VIEWS OF MENTORING: A NEW PARADIGM

It is evident that women are inventing a new paradigm of mentorship. Female mentoring is different from the male mentor model. This new paradigm is reflective of a new world view and a new value system of helping others. It is natural that the face of mentoring among women will have a different look, in the same way that research has delineated differences between men and women's life experiences and preferred styles and approaches to moral decision making, learning, and leading. Since the 1960s, as a result of the women's movement and various societal changes, women have redefined justice, education, and leadership as well as family, sexuality, and equality (Astin & Leland, 1991).

The landmark work of Gilligan (1993), for example, alerted us to the difference in the way that women and men make moral decisions. Her studies documented women's central value of maintaining relationships in confronting moral dilemmas. She postulates that maintaining a central focus on "relationship requires a kind of courage and emotional stamina which has long been a strength of women, insufficiently noted and valued." Likewise, education that is sensitive to women's values should include "connected teaching." This relational teaching emphasizes connection over separation, understanding over assessment, and collaboration over debate (Belenky, Clinchy, Goldberger, & Tarule, 1986). Similarly, in the workplace women's evolving role has produced insights into women's ways of leading and following and their preferred styles of leadership. An interactive-inclusive style of leadership emerges most frequently among women managers in contrast to the traditional command-and-control, bureaucratic style. By engaging in an interactive-inclusive leadership style, women encourage participation, share power and information, enhance another's self-worth, and energize others to succeed (Rosener, 1990). Feminine leadership is related to the "affiliative focus," which is defined as an overriding value for responsibility and interconnection, rather than the quest for authority and autonomy (Miller, 1976). The new paradigm leadership, integrating the female ethos, emphasizes relationships, empowerment, and inclusion (Aburdene & Naisbitt, 1992; Helgesen, 1990; Rogers, 1988). It is useful to view this leadership model as not inherently female but as female developed and female led. The new paradigm leadership is grounded in feminine values. Men and women are capable of being both traditional and new paradigm leaders in an evolving, androgynous style (Guido-DiBrito, Noteboom, Nathan, & Fenty, 1996). An investigation of male and female chief executive officers and chief nursing executives found that although they all used transformational leadership to a greater degree than the transactional style, the female executives scored higher on flexibility and connection to others (Borman, 1993). Borman makes the case that if these differences are translated into behaviors, they will be advantageous to women and nurses in rapidly changing and restructured organizations.

In a study of the developmental relationships of nurses within the work context, including personality and professional values, Wright (1992, 1993) indicates that despite a patriarchal health care system that does not value nurses' and women's work, nurturing and caring still remain central to their work. She suggests that nurses have adopted a different paradigm for their developmental relationships, character- ized by the following:

- mutuality and affiliation;
- complexity and ambiguity;
- cooperation versus competition;
- an emphasis on human relations;
- process versus task;
- acceptance of feelings;
- networking versus hierarchy; and
- recognition of the values of intuition.

To illustrate a new paradigm of mentorship, we developed a chart (Table 3.1) that contrasts traditional and new mentorship, the latter being proposed as women's way of mentoring. This chart classifies the major characteristics of the two paradigms. Elements of both para- digms may, of course, be present in any mentor relationship. Elements in each paradigm may also interlap, but for discussion purposes, they are kept separate. The contrasting characteristics of mentorship are indicative of gender-preferred styles and the gender-related experience of mentorship that comes from personal development, career social- ization, and societal roles. Although it is true that women are creating a different model of mentoring, based on their unique development, needs, and perspectives, we believe that the paradigm will evolve into a new pattern—an integration of both world views of mentoring. This evolutionary paradigm will offer a more holistic and fulfilling men- toring experience for both women and men. The new mentorship is an androgynous model. It is characterized by inclusion, diversity, peer-to- peer connections, long-term and cyclic mentoring, affiliation, and empowerment.

EXCLUSION AND INCLUSION

The traditional mentor-protégé dyad consists of an exclusive one-to- one relationship. This dyad was traditionally composed of two men, one older and more experienced than the other. This form of mentor relationship was most visible in hierarchical, male-dominated profes-

TABLE 3.1 Two World Views of Mentoring

Traditional Mentorship	*New Mentorship*
Exclusive	Inclusive
Similar	Diverse
Expert-to-Novice	Peer-to-Peer
Limited Term	Long Term
Ongoing	Cyclic
Competitive	Affiliative
Power	Empowerment

sions and corporations. In contrast, empirical and anecdotal evidence suggests that rather than engaging in an exclusive dyad only, many female professionals experience multiple mentors throughout their careers. The exclusive dyad of one expert-mentor and one novice-protégé is being supplemented by eclectic mentoring that takes into account diverse needs at various developmental points. Nurses have consistently reported the presence of mentoring from a variety of persons, including teachers, work superiors, peer-colleagues, other professionals, friends, and family. These helping relationships reflect the notion of mentoring influences occurring on a continuum—from more formal and professional to that of informal and peer/friendship connections. Today's professional woman also is engaging more frequently in female-to-female mentoring, in addition to having male mentors. Female mentors also are reaching out and becoming available to male protégés. The web of inclusion is manifested by an openness to many kinds of interconnections and bonds.

SIMILARITY AND DIVERSITY

Sameness has been a notable characteristic of classic mentor relationships. The typical mentor-protégé dyadic composition was that of White males. Sameness in the model also was characterized by the mentor always being older and more experienced than the protégé. Historically, men mentored men, creating a line of succession in the professions and the corporate world. The emerging mentor paradigm has a diverse nature. Diversity speaks to the new forms of partnership that account for differences in gender, ethnicity, race, experience, age, and professional focus. Mentor and protégé do not always have to be "look-alikes." Finding mentors who are "different" can create valuable learning experiences and an expansion of perspective.

EXPERT-TO-NOVICE AND PEER-TO-PEER

The traditional hierarchical form of mentorship is characterized by an older, more experienced, mentor providing advice and guidance to a younger, inexperienced protégé. In contrast, peer-collegial mentor relationships are frequently reported by women and nurses. It is increasingly clear that peers are able to provide similar functions as traditional mentors (Kram & Isabella, 1985), which is an important issue for women in the light of the scarcity of traditional mentors for them. Peer-to-peer mentoring, which figures so prominently in the paradigm, reminds us that mentors do not always have to be the most powerful people. Although work superiors, teachers, specialists, and leaders play a significant role in professional development, particularly at earlier career stages, peers are pivotal mentors throughout our lives. Furthermore, if they are same-gender peers, they serve as important identification figures and role models. A strong and lasting sense of colleagueship develops from the sharing and learning that occurs among peers who are literally living "in the same boat." Peers can identify with and model for each other.

LIMITED AND LONG-TERM MENTORING

Traditional mentor-protégé relationships among men reportedly last for 2 to 3 years (8 to 10 years at the most) and end abruptly, frequently over a competitive issue or when the protégé completes his studies. Mentoring relationships among women and nurses often endure over long periods of time, through many cycles of change and growth. They frequently evolve into collegial collaboration and friendships, and only end in a long-distance move or death. In interviews with the nurse-influentials, many dyads reported long-term relationships. Some of these flourished for 30 to 40 years, with an average length of 15 years. Subsequent studies of nurses' mentoring continue to confirm this trend of abiding relationships.

ONGING AND CYCLIC

Classic mentoring implies a single intense relationship that goes on for a limited period of time and then is ended. In contrast, many nurses report cycles or series of mentoring relationships. These relationships are activated, either as mentor or protégé, at various turning points in their careers. Many women find value in having different mentors for different reasons and in different seasons of their lives. The emphasis on the type of help sought changes from year to year. Career decision points are probably the most delicate ones in the mentor-protégé relationship, because they usually imply new emphases and new phases in the relationship.

COMPETITIVE AND AFFILIATIVE

The evolving model of mentorship postulates that affiliations and attachments are a central element, in contrast to the male model that is frequently characterized by competition and power. Although some degree of competitiveness is present in relationships, through their value for interconnectedness and responsibility for each other, historically women have bonded together for sharing and supporting each other. The power and control factor in mentoring relationships among nurses, however, has been documented (Holloran, 1989, 1993) and should continue to be explored. Collaborative mentorships with doctoral nursing students that celebrate affiliation and diversity of life experience, culture, world view, thought, practice, and method have been postulated as a model in the profession (Meleis, Hall, & Stevens, 1994). The authors promote the activation of this nontraditional mode of mentorship. The features of this collaborative mentorship are negotiated relations, mutual interactions, facilitative strategies, and empowerment, and also incorporate principles of feminist pedagogy.

POWER AND EMPOWERMENT

Power and authority, by virtue of position and background, often hold sway in traditional mentor relationships. Studies of women and nursing leaders continue to illustrate the empowering nature of their mentoring activities. They share with and invest power in their protégés and colleagues, and this sharing becomes a source of their own power. Empowerment is considered a major attribute of women's leadership, and empowerment is a distinct feature of women's mentorship. Empowerment is believing in and encouraging people to access their own power. It is not power *over*, but power *with*. Empowerment is a partnership of sharing that enhances both the power of others and oneself (Surrey, 1991). One study reported that female leaders who were social activists and change agents empowered others by deliberately mentoring them. By empowering others, these leaders were able to create a collective network that has played an ongoing role in transforming institutions (Astin & Leland, 1991).

ISSUES IN FEMALE MENTORING

Mentoring is a compelling concept for today's professional woman. It is increasingly clear that mentor relationships, as well as mentoring activities with various kinds of support persons, are necessary for women's full personal and professional development. Because of their values, developmental issues, and actual experiences, women should be able to engage in mentoring easily. It has been suggested that a framework of reciprocity, empowerment, and solidarity underlies feminist views of mentoring (DeMarco, 1993). The case for the natural affinity of women to be mentors and protégés for reciprocal empowerment and solidarity is poignantly stated by Miller (1991): "I think most women would be most comfortable in a world in which we feel we are not limiting, but are enhancing the power of other people while simultaneously increasing our own power." Mentoring suggests a cooperative, facilitative, caring relationship in which power is shared and mutual benefits are realized. Women intuitively have a great yearning for involvement in such relationships. Interviews with influential leaders in nursing reveal their willingness and sense of responsibility in helping and supporting others. The unique contributions of women mentoring women are expressed in the voices of several of these leaders (Vance, 1986)

> "Your work life, your professional and personal life, everything you do is much more fitting to the woman on the way up than it is from a man whose experiences and outlook are so different. . . . You can much more directly model your behavior on women because you're more like another woman. All of it—all of women's experiences, in whatever area—is very, very useful."
>
> "Modeling and support by a woman are important. Male and female experiences differ, and how women do things may be different from men. I think it's important for a woman who has entered that network and survived, to facilitate and show another woman what it's all about—how to survive and grow in a very paternalistic system."
>
> "The unique benefit to women mentoring women is role

modeling. How can a man model for a woman? In general, nobody will help a woman like another woman."

"From where I sit as a woman, it looks to me . . . [as if] women are able to achieve more intimacy, more sharing and warmth, without discomfort and anxiety. One of the most important things I do as a mentor is to discuss how one spends time and energy on the role juggling women must do."

"If you have a good mentoring relationship with a woman, there is a collegiality and a sharing that is different than that with a man. The sexual overtones are also not there."

"Women should not be coopted into modeling traditional male achievement patterns. Women mentors may eventually produce in their protégés a group who develop new achievement patterns."

"Women tend to be more sensitive, more in touch with feelings, more process-oriented. We have the potential to use our emotional sensitivity in competitive situations and when challenging others' ideas."

"An important thing for women in the mentor relationship is that women have a great need to know that it's O.K. to be yourself. To get that message from another woman is really important. So there is real merit for younger women working with women who have 'made it'—there's something very positive about seeing that another woman has done it—it shows it's possible."

"Women's experiences ought to help women. If you haven't encountered certain things, it would be difficult to appreciate them. So women can understand and contribute something quite differently than a male mentor."

"I think the future of the world depends on women relating to women differently than they do now. It is tremendously important in nursing for women to be able to move into mature collegial mentoring relationships with one another."

To summarize, for women in this study, the unique benefits of having a woman mentor are:

- sharing mutual understanding and experiences as women;
- role modeling as professional women; and
- creating different success and achievement models in society.

GENERATIONAL MENTORING

It is widely acknowledged that as women have entered and stayed in the workplace, they are creating a generational legacy of mentored colleagues. The nurse-influentials were able to identify the mentors who helped them through 2 decades. At the time of the study, the nurse-influentials were assisting their protégés, many of whom have become current leaders and are mentoring another generation of colleagues and potential leaders. Those who have been mentored usually will mentor others. Nursing leaders demonstrate a distinct line of generational mentorship. Because of their mentor connections, they create webs of influence throughout the profession, providing a link from the present into the future. This is significant and encouraging information for women in all life-career stages. In spite of a lingering unawareness or disbelief that long-term sponsorship of this type occurs in female-dominant professions, nurses are creating among themselves a generational line of mentorship that will ultimately enrich the entire profession.

BARRIERS TO BUILDING MENTOR CONNECTIONS

Notwithstanding the necessity of mentor connections for the contemporary female professional, many obstacles exist for their formation and widespread implementation. These obstacles are of an interpersonal, organizational, and individual nature. The barriers to building mentor connections include: (a) inadequate information; (b) unwillingness to seek help; (c) queen-beeism; (d) oppressed mentality; (e) isolation from informational and professional networks; (f) the "old" leadership approach; (g) scarcity of mentors; (h) time issues; and (i) organizational and professional constraints.

Inadequate information about the mentoring process precludes the desire to seek mentoring help. Those who do not know the importance of mentorship for career success or have not been mentored will not know its value and may not reach out actively for or give this assistance. Some people are *unwilling to seek help* and hesitate to initiate a mentor relationship. Perhaps they believe they should be able to manage on their own, fear being "found out" through their lack of knowledge, or feel unworthy of being helped. *"Queen-beeism"* also has contributed to the scarcity of mentors. The queen bee pulls herself up the professional and leadership ladder, but feels no kinship with other women and makes no attempt to help other women achieve. There also may be a resentment of younger people who have had access to opportunities that senior people did not have. The *mentality of oppression*, characterized by low self-esteem, envy, and distrust, causes women to learn to disaffiliate with each other, to see each other as competitors, and to not offer help or seek help from one another (Roberts, 1983).

It has been suggested that women traditionally have not learned to be good team players, to develop collective strategies for winning, to be trustworthy allies, and to join together for mutual benefits (Hennig & Jardim, 1977). There also continues to be instances of "professional hazing." One can imagine how different the outcomes are, professionally and personally, for neophyte nurses if they are carefully and intentionally mentored rather than "hazed." *Isolation from networks and connections* may occur with those who work in organizations where mentoring is not a core value. Self-imposed isolation also can happen by not joining professional associations or looking for networking opportunities. The *"old" leadership approach* is authoritarian, controlling, and characterized by a command-and-control mode that does not encourage a participative, learning, guiding focus. "Making it on your own" and "not coddling" are organizational tenets that do not lend themselves to mentoring. Mentors may be *scarce* depending on the availability of those who have the commitment and generosity to mentor others. Until recently, there have not been substantial numbers of women in positions of power who have had the networks, knowledge, and skill to be able to offer assistance to others. Those who have been in these positions have frequently found themselves inundated with requests for assistance, and *time* resource issues have become problematic. Mentoring inevitably requires a substantial time and energy commitment. Many people get caught up in their own priorities or too many other priorities that appear more important, or cannot seem to "make the time" to devote to others' development. Various *organizational and professional constraints* may prevent widespread formal and informal mentoring because of philosophical, structural, and cultural barriers. Organizational climate and culture undoubtedly influence the development of mentor connections in the workplace. Some organizations isolate, alienate, and foster competition and dependency, while others emphasize and support employee development and collaborative team behaviors. In these learning organizations, leaders are rewarded for the accomplishment of their team members, and mentoring undoubtedly will be pervasive.

Because of various barriers, informal mentor relationships and formal mentor programs may not occur easily, despite the value of mentoring. When barriers are acknowledged and addressed, individuals and groups who desire mentor relationships can work to overcome these obstacles and create these connections.

PART II

Perspectives on Mentorship

4

Living the Mentor Connection:
Personal Reflections and Stories

A good story is a kind of hologram of the life of an individual, a culture, or a whole species. Each of us hears in it, with ears conditioned by our own history, what we most need at the time to understand (Daloz, 1986).

In an evolving and shifting paradigm of mentorship, different points of view and different voices are emerging. All of these perspectives are valid for the participants in mentor relationships. A growing body of research provides us with important information about mentorship. Storytelling is another way to understand the mentoring phenomenon. Storytelling allows us to create and pass on traditions; preserve the important knowledge, values, and concerns of our culture and our profession; share our ideas, experience, and wisdom; and teach and learn through drawing lessons (Benner, 1984, 1991; Boykin & Schoenhofer, 1991; Heinrich, 1992; Larkin & Zahourek, 1988; Lumby, 1993; Rittman & Sella, 1995; Sandelowski, 1991). Storytelling is fundamental to the human search for meaning, and we help each other invent new kinds of stories as we tell the tales of our experiences, past choices, and present dilemmas (Bateson, 1990).

The stories of nurses' mentor connections can inspire, instruct, and encourage. These narratives contain the legacies and values of our profession. Our voices are a way of connecting with and encouraging each other. They also are a vehicle for creativity and for change and transformation. The stories of mentorship in the profession attest to the spirit—the magic—of mentoring, for *magic* is about what we cannot see, but can experience—that which cannot be contained in theoretical formulations and quantitative studies. DeMarco (1993) suggests that women's lived experiences of mentoring, that is, their reality, should be explored by sharing stories. These narratives provide alternative ways of "knowing" about women's support relationships, life, and work and how they can bring new meaning to each other through these relationships.

The following stories and essays about mentoring provide many different perspectives on the experience of mentorship. These perspectives are both personal and universal. They convey the unique diversity and richness of mentor relationships. Nurses' mentoring stories attest to the influence of these relationships on human growth and development and to their staying power in the participants' lives. The narrators' voices speak of connection and caring that transforms individual lives, the workplace, the profession, and the larger society.

Mentoring: A Song of Power

by Beverly Malone

Mentoring is a type of nurturance. Women have genetically and psychosocially specialized in the art of nurturance. As mothers, we sing songs of love, encouragement, and growth to our children. With songs that state, "I love you a bushel and a peck . . . a bushel and a peck and a hug around the neck," we instill in our children an inner reserve of hope, confidence, and power for meeting their futures. Nursing is a profession established on the solid rock of nurturance. Nursing calls it "caring." We excel at providing nurturance to patients. We must learn to nurture other nurses. As nurses, we must sing songs of power to our potential leaders—songs of advocacy for our most fragile, songs of opportunity when faced with adversity, and songs of empowerment that assure our future leaders that they may be diverted but not defeated. We must sing songs of unity, victory, and celebration as we push inch by inch steadily forward. These songs of power must be sung not only to our protégés but to one another, leader to leader and nurse to nurse.

Mentoring is a song of power that becomes embedded in the very fabric of one's existence. In your darkest night, it is the song that comes to your memory in phrases and smells and sensations speaking of strategies, tactics, and visions of change. It is the song of reassurance that provides reason for one's existence and for choosing to be a nurse in this time in this place. When in doubt, nurses must sing the song of mentoring—the song of hope, power, and direction. The message never changes—always toward the delivery of quality health care to all people. This song of power must be sung to our students at every level of education, to our staff nurses, researchers, administrators, practitioners, and faculty.

LEARNING TO SING THE SONG—A PERSONAL SONG

I first learned to sing the song of mentoring from my Granny. She was 65 when I was born. She taught me songs of healing, the song of laughter, and the song of power. For indeed, she was a healer. "Bevh lay," with a strong, slow Kentucky accent, she would sing, "Go pick that leaf, and over there, get that root." And from the leaves and roots, she would mix a salve that grew hair on a baby's bald head. She stood almost 6 feet tall, with lovely silver hair and the long nose and dramatic facial features of an Indian. Her skin was copper, and she told me that her hair had been red when she was young, the daughter of a slave and a White master. Granny organized my world. She taught me to read from the Bible by the time I was 4. Friends and visitors were expected to bring me books to read, or they were not truly welcome in Granny's house. With limited resources, she effectively positioned my world for me to succeed. As I watched this elderly, agile woman wield power and authority, I treasured her songs of endurance and creativity. She was a matriarch, a widow who clearly expressed her desire to make her own decisions as well as yours. During my time with her, she raised, housed, fed, and healed more than 30 different people. There was always food enough, room enough, and love enough to include others. Yet I never doubted that I was the center of her life. I received her song of commitment, clearly understanding that more would be required of me. As a business woman, she was too astute to invest so much without demanding maximum return. The cloak of leadership and responsibility would be passed to me. By the time I was 8 years old, Granny was very ill, and over the next several years, our roles were reversed. The cloak of leadership and responsibility came early, but the song of mentoring is with me forever.

Mentoring, Leadership, and Power—the Professional Song

Mentoring and power are inextricably linked by the concept of leadership. While mentoring is part of the preparatory process of leading, power is its execution. Nursing has been unfamiliar with both the concept of power and mentoring, publicly avoiding the shadow of assertive, goal-oriented behaviors that potentially mold and shape others. Although leadership has been a favorite topic in the nursing literature, it is only recently that power and mentoring have entered the nursing arena legitimately. With a quick scan, one may conclude that the delicacy and propriety of the predominantly female nursing profession precluded such deliberately, competitive, male-type behaviors designed to influence and control organizations and groups. Perhaps this is a variable in the matrix that explains nursing's reticence to acknowledge the need for power and mentoring in the development of nursing leaders.

Another perspective is that power has been deliberately packaged to be aversive or inaccessible to women. This argument is easily supported by the term "MEN-tor." The traditional mentor has usually been White, male, and a powerful senior member of the organization. Mentors tend to be attracted to protégés with whom they can identify. As a result, women have found the availability of mentors to be scarce. Nurses, in particular, have found a void of accessible, available mentors in health care organizations. In other words, mentoring has been wrapped in a package that is foreign to nurses. This perspective is not to deny that there are powerful female leaders in nursing. But many of these leaders may suffer from the queen-bee syndrome. This female syndrome is based on a model of the oppressed: There is only one position at the top and only one privileged female can occupy the position at a time; therefore, all other females are viewed as competitors who must be actively or passively eliminated. The withholding of mentoring to potential protégés is passive elimination of contenders for leadership.

The Racial Face of Mentoring and Power—A Song of Color

With these restrictive leadership issues for nurses and women, accessibility to mentoring is complicated further by race. Black female nurses are faced with the triple "whammy" of their status as women, nurses, and Blacks, which creates a barrier to accessing mentoring relationships. Since available mentors have historically been males, and even if females, usually White, the stereotypical concepts (e.g., matriarchal, oversexed, incompetent, and unattractive) frequently assigned to Black females may stand as potential obstacles in the establishment of a White male or female mentor/Black female protégé relationship. While Black women have turned to other creative, informal, support networks with subordinates, peers, their families, churches, and communities, Black female administrators tend to have been formally mentored.

My doctoral dissertation (Malone, 1981) explored the subject of mentoring as it relates to career satisfaction in the lives of Black female administrators in university (private and public) and corporate settings. Approximately one third of the sample were nurses. Of the total sample of 130 Black women, 80% had been mentored. The majority were older than 40, having earned their high school diplomas before they were 18. They were very well educated, with more than 82% prepared at the master's or doctoral level. Perhaps related to their age, 80% had attended all-Black schools during their educational preparation. Most (86%) were married or had been married at some point in their lives and had children. Sixty-four percent attended church at least once a month, and, before the age of 18, 96% had attended church at least once a month. This study revealed a song of deprivation, achievement, and endurance. Perhaps the message is that Black women leaders achieve through endurance and system survival skills acquired through mentoring and family, church, and community support. The lack of mentoring reduces the possibility of leading for Black females. This may be one explanation for 80% of the leadership sample having had mentor relationships. For the most part, those Black females who were not mentored never progressed to leadership roles.

The sad song of deprivation relates to a lack of current mentoring by the majority of these successful Black female administrators. While most were involved in mentoring others, only a few had current, active, intense mentoring relationships for themselves. The majority of the women retained a somewhat distant relationship with their mentors, but most considered themselves to be too successful and too busy to continue to have a viable, highly interactive mentoring relationship. This lack of vital nurturance contributed to the sadness and sense of loss associated with the intensity and support experienced during earlier periods in their careers and lives.

CLOSING THOUGHTS—A SONG OF BEGINNING

Mentoring is a natural, professional nursing activity of caring, empowerment, and nurturance that must be provided nurse to nurse and leader to leader. While mentoring is natural to the profession of nursing, it is a learned behavior that is facilitated by modeling and the lived experience of having a mentor. Schools of nursing must be incubation units for mentoring. Leaders need mentoring environments. The university should be constructed and reengineered as a mentoring institution (Parks, 1992). The song of mentoring needs to shake and shape the walls of the nursing profession to generate leaders for health care and the global community.

Interview of a Teacher-Mentor and Student-Protégé

by Jane K. Bruker and Melissa L. Charlie

This mentor-protégé relationship occurred when Ms. Bruker was chairperson of the associate degree nursing program at the University of New Mexico-Gallup and Ms. Charlie, who is Navajo, was a student in the program. Melissa is now a full-time doctoral student at the University of Pennsylvania.

INTERVIEW WITH JANE K. BRUKER

Q: How did you decide to mentor Melissa?

JKB: That is a rather silly question. I don't believe one can successfully set out to mentor someone. I believe it has to be a mutual arrangement. By that, I mean before a mentor relationship can be established, a trust relationship must be established. A mentor is more than a guide. I had Melissa in my class and recognized her extraordinary ability to think through a challenge. This in itself was a challenge to me: to give her additional problems to solve—to push, to challenge.

Q: You said you had Melissa in class. When was that and how did the relationship build?

JKB: Melissa was a student in our program. I teach the mental health component, and at that time I also was the chairperson of the program. As I said, I had recognized her ability to think through things and her knowledge of many diverse subjects. She also expressed an interest in campus politics. In our program we had the president of the Nursing Student Club as a voting member of our nursing faculty and curriculum committees. Melissa was the president of the club and attended these meetings. She took a very active part and was influential in many of our decisions. Her comments were valued by all faculty. I would have to say, however, that some faculty resented the inclusion of a student as a voting member.

Q: What do you think of present attempts at mentoring?

JKB: I guess I am concerned that it is a buzzword that really will mean nothing unless women understand the need to truly support each other. As I mentioned, some of the faculty resented a student even coming to the faculty meetings, let alone being allowed to argue with and challenge the faculty and to vote. Since I was the chairperson of the program, I could include Melissa. If I had been a faculty member, I might not have had the support. I have seen other attempts at mentoring fail because of this lack of understanding or even fear that a younger, perhaps more enthusiastic, intelligent person is being introduced to the "inner sanctum." I am afraid that women may be more inclined to this fear than men.

Q: Was there a turning point or specific time that you became a mentor and not just a teacher?

JKB: On one occasion, I asked the class what their professional goals were. The class had the usual responses, such as work in pediatrics, the emergency room, and so on. Melissa, however, responded with, "I want your job." I thought that was great and decided to give her whatever help I could to help her reach that goal.

Q: What kind of help did you give?

JKB: I believe that I have been fairly successful as a program chairperson. I also have been very active in nursing organizations. I believe that to be a true change agent, that is, to effectively make changes in the delivery of health care, it must be done through nursing education, nursing service, and the nursing organizations working together. Since I have been in nursing for over 40 years, I have seen many times when quarreling or back-stabbing hurt not only individuals but the entire profession. I have seen so-called leaders in nursing keep such a tight rein and control on their organizations as to stifle the growth of any of the members. I wanted Melissa to have the opportunity to grow for herself, but also to see some of the negative things that occur in the professional realm, so that she would be better able to evaluate roles and decisions.

Q: Were there some stressful periods of learning?

JKB: There were many times when I wondered what my role was. On one occasion when we were talking about how changes to something or other should be made, I said it was necessary to understand politics and to play the political game. Melissa became unglued and shouted that she would not compromise her beliefs, and if people wanted to change they would have to listen to her because she knew what it was like to be a minority and I didn't. Of course, her statement was correct—she belongs to a minority group, and I do not. My challenge was how I could help her to understand that I was not telling her that she had to become "White" or deny her ethnicity, but that she did have to listen to other people to be able to counter their arguments. She went through much agony about what exactly is meant by "playing the political game." I believe she finally realized that it does not mean changing your mind or being shallow or deceitful, but it does mean listening to your constituents, whoever they may be (other students, faculty, or nurses).

Q: What did you do that you believe was the most beneficial in Melissa's learning?

JKB: There were three major things that I did that I believe were very helpful. The first was including her in faculty meetings and taking her to meetings of every kind with me. I did not specify to her what her role should be. I suggested she might want to talk to this person or that, or that she might want to attend this meeting or that, but what she did was really up to her. By that, I mean, I gave her the opportunity, and it was up to her to take advantage of it. I think this is extremely important in any mentoring relationship. It is probably something that should be examined carefully when we look at mentor relationships with women.

Because women tend to want to have the mothering or protecting role, growth may not take place at an internal level because the change is imposed upon, rather than internalized. The second thing was to encourage her to attend a school that was in a different part of the country. It was difficult for me because it meant that I would not have the same influence on her that I had enjoyed previously. However, I believe it is very important in our present mobile world that people learn and experience learning in a variety of settings and that this was critical to her education. The third thing is understanding that, although the original idea was that she would take my job, as she grows and her opportunity and experience expand, she may want other things. Included in this is that I have had to recognize from the beginning that she might, and in all probability will, exceed me in both educational and professional accomplishments. It is important that I take this as a compliment to my tutelage and not as a threat to my importance.

Q: Do you think Melissa feels the mentor relationship has been in her best interest?

JKB: I cannot know what her feelings are about that. I know that she has had the opportunity to discuss her ideas with other people. She has not been tied to this campus, for example. I think that is an important part of the relationship. If the mentor has the power of giving a grade or a promotion or even a recommendation for a job, the freedom for growth is diminished. It must be a totally free learning environment. That is why I question what we sometimes call "mentors." I believe the mentor concept in the classroom is more a guided learning or an individualized teaching experience, not a true mentorship. I also do not believe mentors can be assigned. It has been suggested that we develop a Mentor Program where we assign minority nurses in the community as mentors to our students. I am not questioning the value of such a scheme; I am questioning the use of the term "mentor."

INTERVIEW WITH MELISSA L. CHARLIE

Q: How would you describe your "mentor connection" with Ms. Bruker?

MLC: In thinking about my mentoring relationship with Jane Bruker, I have a mental picture of Jane opening a door for me. At times, it felt as if she had to push me through the door, but eventually, I journeyed to a different place, and I shall never be the same again. I first met Jane in April 1990. In the years that followed, what set Jane apart from other people who had *told* me that I had potential was that she *treated* me as if I had potential. Plenty of teachers and professors told me that I was smart, intelligent, and capable, but that was the extent of their interest in my potential. Along with that, she also treated me like an equal. I felt that my voice was as important as that of other faculty members. She challenged me from the beginning, and I liked that. Her actions said to me that she thought I am as intelligent as she is. Being treated like an equal was a new experience for me. In my educational experience, I always felt that teachers and professors had to defend their turf and that the faculty felt that they had to be more "right" than the students, always. Now I had Jane treating me as if I had as much insight into the problems of the community as she did. I was the expert on what it feels like to grow up in the unique community of Gallup, and Jane relied on me to gain insight into possible educational solutions to some of the community problems, and to assist in decision making.

Q: How did you decide to let Jane be your mentor?

MLC: I didn't really decide to let Jane mentor me. In fact, I don't think I would label our relationship as a "mentor" relationship. I think of mentoring as hierarchical in nature, meaning that the person with all the knowledge and experience gives to the person without the knowledge and experience. In contrast, in my relationship with Jane, I have always felt that we were equals and that we learned from each other. In fact, if Jane had not treated me like an equal, I would not have developed the kind of relationship that we have. Growing up Navajo in Gallup, New Mexico, left me hypersensitive to inequality. When I first met Jane, I was so young and impatient that I could not stand to be in the presence of anyone who had a condescending attitude toward Indians. I felt such rage that all I could do was walk away. Jane never treated me as if she knew so much more about the world than I did.

Q: What things have you learned from Jane?

MLC: Well, I think I can say that my relationship with Jane has left me with three wonderful strengths. I do not say that she gave me these strengths because I had to do the work to get them, but I do give her all the credit for taking the time to germinate and to nurture those strengths and to have the vision to see those strengths when they were not yet there. The first strength I grew with Jane is the ability to create change. Never before had I felt that my words, my ideas, and my actions could create change. I saw that when I spoke at the curriculum meetings, the faculty and Jane listened and occasionally acted on my ideas. I saw myself changing the emotional environment of the student nurses by being politically active on campus. The second strength Jane and I grew was the ability to see the world from a very different perspective. I grew up in an environment very different from Jane's. Age alone does not explain that difference. She grew up in a very solid family, very educated, and what I would call classic white Anglo-Saxon Protestant. She had more money than I ever had. I grew up in a single-parent family, not economically stable, and not educated. When I first met Jane, I almost could not believe that she had ever felt sadness in her life. In my experience, she had none of the things that cause sadness. As I told Jane about the difficulty of growing up as I did, like many people in our area do, she understood me but in a different context. And I learned that there are many ways people feel constrained, feel pain, or feel "less than." Even though I knew that White people are not all alike and that everyone feels pain for different reasons, I had never experienced that in a relationship before. This experience helped me get rid of a lot of bitterness and resentment that I had had about growing up poor, and about being treated as less than others. The third strength that Jane and I grew, that she gently helps me grow, is the strength to admit error. At one point, I told Jane that I could never be nice to someone I didn't like, and that essentially, I could not play the political game. I was wrong about that. I learned to see that some goals are worth fighting for and that if I did not work to change things with whatever means ethically possible, I would not be doing all that I could do. I used to think that appearances did not matter. I was wrong about that. As a friend said to me, "It is important to be careful of who you appear to be."

Q: What do you think of present attempts at mentoring?

MLC: I think that "mentor" is an overused word, generally used to describe almost anyone who gives support to a student. Consequently, I don't think it is possible to assign a student to a specific mentor. I don't believe it is possible to tell someone, "This is your mentor." Yet, in assigning a student to a mentor, that is what one is saying. One can assign a student to a resource person, but not to a mentor. Currently I am a doctoral student and on the nursing faculty at the University of New Mexico-Gallup. One of the things that I think about is how to make myself open to being someone's mentor. There are "things" that Jane did to make herself more open to me. What are those "things?" Jane has taught me how to be a role model, but not how to be a mentor. The issue is, how do nurses make themselves more available to become mentors?

Q: What do you think of your mentor relationship?

MLC: Jane Bruker is the first person who honestly believed in my potential. By her actions, I felt and knew she believed in me. When I tried to get information from universities across the country about R.N.-M.S.N. programs, Jane called people she knew at different universities. When some of those universities told us that they did not want an associate degree student, Jane called the dean of the College of Nursing at Syracuse University and asked her to recruit me. When I was immobile with self-doubt, Jane made me sit at a desk for hours until I finished my application to Syracuse University. Even though I was kicking and screaming, Jane pulled me through that first door of success. That is all I needed. Ever since then, I have known my direction in life and have followed it, despite obstacles.

JKB and MLC: We believe that a mentor relationship is a serious commitment for an indeterminate period of time. It must allow for flexibility on the part of the mentor, and the mentor's predetermined goals and personal objectives for the protégé have to be set aside. The only long-range goal is that the protégé will have an opportunity to reach her potential. There has to be a commonality, not specific goals and objectives, but a desire to make change.

Mentorship: A Personal Perspective

by Marla E. Salmon

Dear Colleague,

When I began to reflect on mentorship, I thought it would be an easy task since I have received tremendous help from my mentors. I soon realized that mentorship is a very personal and individual experience; thus I am writing my thoughts as an open letter to you, the reader. In my mind, you are someone who might be grappling with the difficult task of making the right choices in your own life—career, relationships, and family. It is my hope that this letter will provide some insights and the knowledge that mentorship is tangible, and that you should see yourself as a participant in it—now as protégé and later as mentor.

On to my own experiences. When I look back on my career, I see the "fingerprints" of many people who shaped it along the way. Were they mentors? Yes, but perhaps not in the conventional sense. Let me explain. Mentorship has come to me in many forms. For many professionals, a mentor is seen as someone in the profession who develops a long-term "bond" with a more junior colleague and helps him or her along the professional journey. In this version of mentorship, the protégé imagines his or her future personified by the mentor. At its most extreme, the protégé's role is to become "like" the mentor—to emulate and imitate. For me, mentorship never worked that way. My mentors were sometimes "of" my profession; however, frequently, they were people whose work was not nursing. Among those I consider to be my mentors, there is a German professor, a political scientist, a zoologist, a community organizer, and a lawyer. All of these people were very important to me. However, they weren't overall professional role models. Indeed, I'm not sure I've actually met someone who could be that. What my mentors shared with me was wisdom, encouragement, and expert knowledge. They modeled approaches, strategies, and behaviors that related to their expertise and experience. One could say that my mentors came in "different seasons for different reasons." Most of my mentorship experiences lasted only a short time—the friendships and colleagueships that grew out of them, however, continue on today. While each of my mentors was different from the others, they all had something in common: they shared commitments and concerns that I had. And, perhaps most important of all, they saw in me a unique potential that they could help to develop. They did not view me as someone who would become like them. They cared about who I was and who I could become. Their efforts were aimed at enabling me to fulfill my own potential.

So, what do my experiences with mentorship mean to you as you move through the stages of your career? First, and most important, they should encourage you to look at your career as the means through which you do something good and worthwhile that you care about—rather than as the path for getting to a certain position or achieving prestige. This approach, however, precludes the tidy career planning method of setting clear, detailed goals and objectives aimed at some ultimate "magic" job. When one actually identifies and clarifies one's own commitments and measures success by how much difference one makes, the task of career planning becomes highly complicated, disorderly, and confusing. It is a bit like being cast about in a dark sea with a distant lighthouse barely in sight. Navigation of these waters is not easy! Before I talk further about navigating career development, however, I want to be very clear about what a career based on commitment means over the course of a lifetime. For me, it has meant a deep satisfaction in knowing that in some ways I have made the world a better place for other people—and that my career has made this possible. It also has meant, however, being haunted by the enormous task of trying to make things better. As a result, making good career choices has been very complex. I have had to rely heavily on others to assist me.

So, how does one effectively plan a commitment-based career, given its complexity? The answer really lies in finding people who can help—those who can provide coaching, modeling, wisdom, and guidance. In other words, if you don't have a well-charted course, then you need to find people who have traveled the waters in which you find yourself and ask for their help in guiding the way. Finding such people is not so difficult—I suspect that you know people around you who share your commitments and concerns and whose work relates to these. Getting them to serve as mentors is not as easy. Although there is no recipe, let me share some observations about what seems to work in this regard.

First, understand that mentorship that is based on shared commitments and concerns is *mutually* rewarding. In other words, the protégé not only receives, but also gives back a great deal to the mentor. The "payoff," of course, is not monetary or related to status. Rather, it lies in the abiding satisfaction of knowing that the mentor relationship has enabled another person to contribute to what you and the mentor care about. Thus when you seek mentorship, you should recognize that what you give back is your future work toward the values and commitments that you share. A true mentor is delighted to see you grow and surpass him or her in your work. Second, understand that a mentor is giving to you in ways that go well beyond the confines of his or her job. This means that you, too, need to function beyond the standard expectations. Mentorship is "extra" work on both sides. You must be prepared to accept demands and expectations that are different from those others may be experiencing. It is this extra investment of all persons that makes mentorship rewarding and worthwhile.

Given these dynamics of mentorship, how does one get it under way? Let's assume that you have someone in mind to serve as a mentor. The next step is for you to simply ask. It is amazing to me how many people are reluctant to approach someone and ask for their insights and assistance. The likelihood of receiving the help you seek is actually enhanced by your demonstrated sincerity and commitment. In other words, the simple act of asking for mentoring is the first concrete indication to your prospective mentor that you want to work toward the commitments that you mutually share. I can guarantee that asking gets easier over time, but do plan to ask many times through the course of your career. Mentorship is something that has lasting value across one's entire career. As such, one must be well attuned to one's own needs for mentoring and the opportunities to seek it. Once you have asked and succeeded in beginning the mentorship process, you will find that there are no recipes for how to proceed from there. This is not a problem, however, because you are no longer alone—you are working with someone who will be your partner in finding these and other answers. One suggestion, though, is to communicate carefully with your mentor. Communication is the very essence of mentorship. Express your interests, ideas, and needs. Also, it is equally important to listen, clarify, and appreciate openly. Mentors are people who have much to give. However, they also need the same attention, feedback, and appreciation as everyone else. As you work with your mentors, you will discover that the fuel that drives mentorship is faith and trust. From its inception, mentorship is a unique human relationship. For both the mentor and the protégé, the relationship is initially built almost entirely on potential and hope rather than "performance." This means that mentorship is grounded in the future rather than the present or past. It is not the kind of relationship that is comfortable for those who need security or assurances. Operating on faith and trust can some-times be a fairly difficult task.

I think that you will find joy and challenge in the mentorship experience. Please recognize, however, that you should never see yourself only in the protégé role. To be a successful protégé, you must also see yourself as a mentor for others. As you are men-tored, you are learning to mentor. In some sense, it is like leader-ship—you must learn to both lead and follow. And, ultimately, to be good at either, you must be competent in performing both roles. Mentorship is a gift. However, it is one that is never truly owned. Rather, it is passed from one person to the next, carrying with it very special rewards and responsibilities. I will close this letter to you by wishing you the very best in your own mentor-ship experiences. You have much to look forward to, and much to do! Bon voyage!

Sincerely yours,
Marla E. Salmon, ScD, RN, FAAN

On Mentoring: A Skeptic's View

by Barbara Stevens Barnum

Mentoring is a word of which I'm leery because so many people use it incorrectly—wrong by my definition, that is. Let me give you an example. Once after I gave a speech somewhere, a woman that I did not recognize came up to talk with me. She introduced herself and thanked me profusely for making it possible for her to achieve her life's goals. I smiled and shook her hand, which was all I could do while I strained for some memory of her. The memory did not come, but, fortunately, she went on with her tale. I would remember, she said, that she came to me for advice when everyone else was telling her that her study plan was impossible. She wanted to do a Ph.D. that virtually combined two complex and difficult majors from two different departments (one was nursing). Both her adviser and the chairman of the other depart-ment said that it couldn't be done and that she was foolish to contemplate doing such extensive work. How she came to me I'll never recall, but apparently I advised her that anything was pos-sible if she was willing to pay the price. I told her to switch advis-ers, indicating which faculty member she should seek in the nursing department and also the faculty member she should approach in the other department. She had followed my advice and now possessed exactly the credentials she had sought. The woman gave me a big hug and said, "Thank you for being the most important mentor in my life." I smiled again and wished her well. I held back the lecture on my tongue—namely, that I wasn't her mentor, just someone who had offered some advice along the way.

There are several points to be made in this story. Teachers who just teach and advise, not to mention good friends or strangers who do the same, may have a pivotal influence on one's life. For all I know, the extensive information I gave a little old lady who asked for directions yesterday may have created a diversion just long enough to stop her from stepping out in front of an approaching bus! Message: While mentoring is important in one's life, other helping relationships are also important. I have had thousands of students in my career. I hope I have helped them all, but I have been mentor to only a few of them. Mentorship, in my conception, is a lifelong relationship in which one person provides not only education and advice but is in a position to serve as a role model as well. To qualify as a mentor, in my view, the person also must be instrumental in providing career opportunities for the other. When we nurses do it, it's mentorship, and we approve. When businessmen do it, we call it the "old boys' network" and turn up our noses. The fact is that, by any terminology, mentoring makes the world go around. Mentoring is an interesting phenomenon often portrayed as the beneficence of the master bestowed for the price of some affective reward. The image isn't right. Trust me, for plain old affective rewards, it's easier to feed off the adulation of a class of students or off incidents such as the one I described earlier in this essay.

Mentorships don't always involve ego stroking, although strong friendships often develop. If the relationship is a good one, the friendship develops for other reasons than its expert and apprentice aspects. Mentorships, by their exclusive nature, are selfish arrangements on both parts. Both parties share in the relationship's successes and failures. Mentorships can, alas, go sour. Sometimes mentors perceive that they were used as stepping stones only to be discarded once the desired upward mobility was achieved. Sometimes, worse, an insecure protégé may feel a need not merely to discard a mentor but also to "put down" the mentor rather than acknowledge the debt. On the other hand, some protégés have found themselves cast in roles akin to galley slaves, relationships in which they are expected to serve as willing subordinates forever rather than find their own independence, not to mention stardom. The benefits are easy to see for the one being mentored, but often masked for the mentor. Yet it is to the mentor's credit (in the larger nursing network) to have protégés that can be recommended when she is asked for assistance in filling positions, picking speakers, looking for committee members, and so on. To have no recommendations marks one as out of the loop. Moreover, having protégés keeps mentors on their toes. Perhaps the protégé's questions make a mentor think through an issue in depth, for example, resulting in a published paper that would not have come about otherwise. So mentorships always work two ways.

Mentoring, as opposed to cronyism, has a teacher-student quality in that the more experienced person not only fosters the other person's career development, but usually teaches him or her something along the way. Unlike the formal educational situation, the teaching tends to be of the apprenticeship/role-modeling sort. Most often, the less experienced person is somewhere "under" the mentor in an organizational arrangement, at least for the early part of their relationship. In this context the protégé comes to rely on the mentor for advice even after their careers have separated and taken different paths. The mentor tends to create opportunities for the protégé over the lifetime of his or her career.

I think the most unlikely mentorship is one to arise between teacher and student, unless that student is learning to be a teacher. That's because the relationship involves a lot of role modeling. And I'm not sure that a teacher can demonstrate the values, work patterns, and type of commitment required of the practitioner. After all, she didn't elect to be one, did she? Most of my protégés have been in nursing service administration simply because that's where I've spent much of my career. Few of them were my students in the traditional sense. This is not to say that I haven't on occasion been assistive to former students. But I'm hesitant to call these relationships true mentorships. You simply can't tell how a person will work in the world from his or her performance in the student role. And if anything marks the protégé, it's that he or she has the mentor's "seal of approval" as competent in a defined role. An interesting point about what one teaches as a mentor: I have always found that only the best people do this form of promoting the next generation. Self-absorbed and weak people can't mentor because they withhold. A good mentor is willing to teach everything she knows (not that she can prevent the protégé from learning by observation in any case).

Some mentors fear being replaced by the protégé or fear that the protégé eventually will be better than they are. So they reveal "some" of their stuff, carefully husbanding away from sight certain aspects of their performance or knowledge. I believe that the withholding is what destroys the weak, would-be mentor. I have always found that when you teach something to someone else, you learn even more in the very act of conveying that information. In a sense, the fear that one will be surpassed because of what one teaches is flawed reasoning. When one teaches, the protégé learns what is taught and the mentor learns something new. The would-be mentor who withholds is the one who will be surpassed. Self-fulfilling prophecies come to mind here. A good mentor won't even be thinking in those terms.

As for effectiveness, a good mentor recognizes the difference between herself and the protégé—recognizing skills she doesn't have and fostering them too. She never tries to make a carbon copy of herself; instead, she encourages the other person to explore new turf, develop career strengths of his or her own. Protégés should be warned not to try to be someone else—and to avoid, like the plague, the mentor who wants a clone. A mentor who seeks to be imitated is a hazard to one's autonomous development. From the perspective of the mentor, protégés are like extra children, and like children, they should eventually move out. To keep a protégé as one's "second" throughout one's career is deleterious to both parties. I know a few protégés who never came into their own because they spent a lifetime being hired as the second in command every time their mentors took new positions. This is not a mentor/apprentice relationship but a master/slave relationship. In it, only the master will shine; the apprentice probably will be doing much of the work in a short time, but will never be recognized as a moving force. That gets into idolatry and the mentor's needs for adulation. Beware of mentors demanding adoration; the queen-bee syndrome is alive and well, even in some strong nurse leaders. Allowing oneself to be fodder for an appetite that requires constant ego feeding is like choosing the door with the tiger behind it. In the best mentorship, the protégé eventually reaches the stage where he or she can see the flaws in the mentor—and tell the mentor. *Full reciprocity is the ideal outcome of a mentorship.* I love it when my protégés tell me they've discovered my flaws and no longer think I'm so "hot."

I never had a mentor in nursing, so I'm certain it's possible to build a career without one. But the right mentorship can make the difference between a slow-developing career and one on a fast track. I had a mentor in my secondary career—philosophy—but I married him and that ended that. (It's poor form to mentor a family member.) Before sacrificing mentorship for marriage, I would suggest you consider where you live. In some towns, it's easier to find a husband than a mentor! That brings us back to affection: Do you have to like each other? I don't think so; the operative word is respect. I really like most of my protégés, but there's at least one for whom I simply can't wrestle up much affection. (Don't tell her, please.) This is a very competent woman whose style, philosophy, and way of managing is totally contradictory to my own—not wrong, you understand, just contradictory. Is that the reason I don't feel much warmth? I don't think so—there are others with radically different approaches of whom I'm extremely fond. In her fashion, she's very good at what she does; for some positions, she is exactly the right choice. I have the greatest respect for her. I'm not convinced that the relationship is poorer for ending there. Some executives consciously strive to create mentor relations. I take a more casual approach: if a relationship develops, it develops. I don't look for it. At least once I had a mentorship relationship forced on me. Her tenacious insistence in the face of my disinterest finally caught my attention and ultimately my respect. Most mentorships develop when a fledgling shows such potential that the would-be mentor can't ignore it. That might happen once or twice in a mentor's career, maybe five or six times if she lives long enough. But when someone tells me she is a mentor to 20 people, I get suspicious. That brings me back full cycle to the meaning of mentorship. In my dictionary, 2 or 3 fledglings make a mentor, 20, a guru. Beware of gurus.

Under the category of best advice for mentors, I've already said most of it: teach everything; withhold nothing; encourage a separate identity; don't become a slave master; eventually kick protégés out of the nest. For the protégé: learn what you can; be grateful but not slavish; don't think you must "kill" the master to succeed; eventually try your own wings.

A Memorable Mentorship

by Virginia Trotter Betts

Mentors, protégés, mentoring—clearly a topic of active discussion in nursing. Yet I find "mentoring" an elusive concept—one that has been more happenstance and a confluence of need and timing rather than a design to further or shape my career. Perhaps as nurses mature in their career orientation away from merely job seeking or job-fulfilling expectations, identifying and seeking appropriate mentors will became as planned for professional nurses as for professionals in corporate America. In thinking of experiences in which I was mentored, they tend to be experiences of the educational type (both formal and informal). They include these criteria:

1. *Need*: My need to learn
2. *Identification*: A positive interpersonal bonding that reflects identification and mutual respect
3. *Facilitation*: A willingness on the part of the mentor to be a colleague and a facilitator, not an authority figure (or a "boss")
4. *Expectations*: An expectation on the part of the mentor to turn over some portion of work to me fully and with responsibility for its outcome

I have had more parent-child, teacher-pupil, expert-novice, boss-staff experiences than mentoring ones. These were characterized by hierarchies, control and authority issues, expectations of compliance to the teacher's prescription, and, if the relationship was extended, eventual competition between the parties. I gained a lot from many of these traditional teacher-pupil relationships, but I learned, valued, and *loved* my mentoring ones. The most memorable mentoring experience of my career occurred the year I spent as a Robert Wood Johnson Health Policy Fellow. The Robert Wood Johnson program has been ongoing for more than 20 years, having as its primary purpose the bringing of health expertise to policy makers in Washington to enhance the substantive content of federal health policy, and providing to universities faculty members who have experiential expertise in federal policy making. Each year the program has a small group of Fellows chosen in a highly competitive process who learn together as a group before "practicing" their knowledge and skills in a federal office.

Since each Fellow chooses and negotiates her or his own federal "assignment," there is almost no way for Robert Wood Johnson program faculty to prepare one for the particular expectations of the chosen assignment. Thus with much knowledge about professional nursing, mental health, and health care law, but very little knowledge of what a Senate staffer really *does*, I joined the office of then Senator Albert Gore as a health legislative assistant. I had a *big* need to learn, and luckily I found a mentor (Criterion 1). My Robert Wood Johnson mentor was Roy Neel. He had been Senator Gore's legislative director for some time and was elevated to administrative assistant, the highest staffer job in a senator's office, just before I arrived. We had much in common—both pushing 40 in an office of 20- and 30-year-olds, Tennesseans, married with children, Vanderbilt graduates, yet still sports enthusiasts. We also loved to work, laughed easily, believed that public policy *can* better people's lives, and were always great pragmatists. We also shared admiration and respect for Senator Gore and his agenda of service for America (Criterion 2). In my relationship with Roy, he paid attention to my work and gave me guidance and feedback rather than criticism (Criterion 3). In fact, when my first briefing memo was requested by the senator, Roy took me aside and showed me examples of his work before I did my first draft. He offered to look over the draft; he made excellent suggestions; and then told me to "put it to bed— no time for perfection here!"

Robert Wood Johnson Fellows bring much to the offices in which they serve, but they also can breed anxiety and competition among other staffers who have less freedom to experiment or who may feel threatened by new expertise. Roy sensed this accurately when it happened in our office, and he swiftly facilitated complementary roles, responsibilities, and tasks that enhanced my learning while preventing "office politics" from limiting my enthusiasm and effectiveness. As the quality of my work and my ability to contribute to the whole of the office became increasingly recognizable, the fourth criterion emerged. I started off working in partnership with an experienced staffer, but, over time, my responsibilities grew to manage a whole issue alone (Criterion 4). In that context I became a significant part of the office and its work—not a "temp" on a short assignment.

When my tenure drew to a close, recognition and appreciation were verbalized by Roy and the senator with an emphasis on my primary contributions as a part of the whole and as a principal for outcomes, not just a support person.

The pattern and criteria I have described are present in my other mentoring relationships as a protégé: need, identification, facilitation, expectations. I have experienced them in many settings. Yet when I reflect on the flip side as mentor, I understand it less because mentoring, I believe, is so personal for the protégé. However, I do worry that so many former students, colleagues, and nurses I meet in many forums frequently ask me career-building questions that focus on my degree in law. I have spent my entire work life as a nurse, and I "happen" to have a law degree and a license. Yet I sense that if I am assertive, articulate, or successful in achieving outcomes for nursing, many folks (potential protégés) prioritize my law degree. I find that troubling because I believe the essence of any professional success I have achieved includes: (a) the analytical problem-solving mode of nursing; (b) the understanding of people and their needs and behavior honed by years of mental health nursing interventions; and (c) the leadership and collectivity skills that have been forged as a result of 2 decades of progressive, professional nursing association involvement. Nursing is a wonderful basis for a career and a life of activism for positive social change. I want my profession—nursing—to be acknowledged and admired by all with whom I come in contact, especially by those who are already committed to the discipline. Are you looking for a mentor? Look to the leaders in the various nursing associations. They are committed to nursing and to a better society. They are excellent potential mentors for your personal and professional growth.

Tapping into Uncommon Wisdom through Mentorship

by JoEllen Koerner

The pursuit of wisdom and mastery, "the mysterious process during which what is at first difficult becomes progressively easier and more pleasurable through practice" (Leonard, 1992, p. xi) is a lifelong journey. The sojourner on this path toward excellence is often found exploring uncharted territory, sometimes going beyond the limits of current understanding, trying to push those

limits outward into new areas. The learning curve is vastly facilitated by exposure to those who display mastery, those who possess uncommon wisdom in the area of inquiry. The physics
principle of induction references the transfer of organized energy
from one system to another (Koerner & McWhinney, 1995). In the
purest sense, induction is achieved by imitation as the mentor
progressively draws the protégé into new patterns through a
rhythm of taking in and letting go (or giving back). A common
psychological model of induction is seen in a parent encouraging
his or her child to walk: the smile—and the countersmile. With
each cycle of response, the pattern of induction becomes more
deeply etched in the protégé's system. All human interactions are
inductive, as in a dance; all are rhythmic exchanges that organize
the energy in each of the exchanging elements.

A conscious commitment to an inductive relationship
through mentoring has enormous potential for mutual enrichment and benefit. In the long run, the profession also is enhanced
because the end result of the mentorship process—a competent
senior professional—is the mentor of the future. Many factors
influence career decisions, patterns of development, and levels of
aspiration. A factor that contributes to keeping many nurses in
midlevel jobs is the lack of a long-term and constant socialization
process that expands career vision and development. A wise and
seasoned mentor provides protégés with support, direction, and
feedback regarding their interpersonal development and career
plans. Thus mentoring occurs when two people choose to engage
in this type of relationship in an environment that supports their
interaction.

Contributions of a Wisdom Keeper to the Mentoring Experience

Evolving professionals create a learning experience with someone, or several persons, who demonstrate wisdom (which is a
"knowing" beyond technical proficiency) in a personal characteristic or skill the protégé desires. For maturing career professionals, research suggests that inductive patterning is not one of
complete imitation of the master as with a novice practitioner, but
that the protégé is highly selective in adopting certain mentor
characteristics that meet his or her immediate needs (Carmin,
1988; Cotton, 1992; Olson, Gresley, & Heater, 1984; Vance, 1982;

Yoder, 1990). Bucher and Steeling (1977) identified three types of role-modeling processes: *partial, stage,* and *option.* In the *partial role-modeling* process, the protégé selects desired attributes from several different mentors. Attributes are chosen that are regarded as compatible with one's sense of self and the projected professional image. Thus the protégé is able to construct an "ideal" professional self from the various mentors available. In *stage modeling,* the protégé seeks more advanced colleagues as information sources concerning future periods of personal and career development. The wisdom keeper is in a mature stage of professional experience and can provide the protégé with tested advice on how to avoid certain difficulties or how to achieve similar success. In *option modeling,* the protégé seeks a mentor with an unusual or deviant career pattern. Career histories that are different from the standard are useful because they give newcomers evidence that alternatives and variations are possible despite the prevalence of the status quo.

Irrespective of which role-modeling process is adopted, the wisdom keeper is vital to the protégé for patterning a professional image compatible with self-perception and professional expectation. The mature mentor may provide the protégé with standards of behavior and professional activity of outstanding leadership: interaction with colleagues and subordinates; conflict resolution and political savvy; balance of personal life and professional demands; ethical decision making; and executive leadership skills in integrative systems. The protégé may be interested in acquiring specific skills in areas of creativity, reflection, or personal awareness that would lead to selection of a different kind of mentor. Or the protégé may be interested in studying career advancement patterns and histories of professional achievement that would take him or her down another path. Any area of study in the realm of personal and professional development is an appropriate focus for the protégé.

CONSIDERATIONS IN SELECTING A WISDOM KEEPER

Factors to consider in selecting a mentor include: the protégé being clear on what is being sought at this point in his or her career; the mentor's demonstrated interest in the protégé's professional development; and a similar or shared value system. There are times in one's development when specific exposure and opportunities are needed to create a "lived experience" from which to draw on. These moments are critical to an expansion of awareness of "what is real." By walking, talking, and reflecting with a mature mentor, the protégé begins to create a memory bank that guides his or her: (a) frame of reference (scope of the issue and number of players involved); (b) sense of importance (is this the "hill to die on?" or is this a perennial issue to be incorporated into a larger strategy, saving the energy for a broader issue?); (c) sense of timing (how ready is the organization or team or individual to move to this new place? . . . how far can the leader go without losing support or momentum?); and (d) deployment of resources (who gets what, why do they get it, in what form would it be most useful, and when should it be made available?). Issues like this can be tested only in the laboratory of actual life experience. Thus a protégé would do well to seek experiences with individuals or organizations involved in issues that are similar in scope (though not necessarily in the same field) to the concepts being sought.

A second kind of "knowing" also is needed, and not as often addressed in plans for personal and professional development. Professional nursing—in all its various domains (clinical, academic, or administrative)—is at its core a function of relationship. Transformative nursing—healing, teaching, and leading—requires the practitioner to "be" the message we espouse. Nurses who reflect the essence of the discipline may be met briefly, but remembered forever. These professionals' lives reflect the essence of healing and wholeness. They attract us because they display the possibility of what our lives might become. We break out of an "oh sure, it's easy for you to be this way" mentality and move to a breathtaking awakening of our own potential (Leegard, 1993). A wisdom keeper is someone walking a path like our own. We listen for words and catch phrases and see a way to follow by walking alongside him or her. We watch the wisdom keeper's movements through the workplace, across his or her careers. It takes time to see and tenderness to hear the message of his or her life journey so we must be attentive to what is happening. Through the example of the wisdom keeper's life manifested in the essence of his or her daily walk, we find guidance for our own.

When I began to grasp the notion and importance of case

management, I searched the field and reviewed the literature, identifying nurse futurists who were testing models and methods around the concept. One name in particular kept emerging, so I called her and made a trip to her state to engage in a dialogue. What began as a conversation and ideas written on the back of a restaurant napkin evolved into a 10-year friendship where the exchange moved in a dialectical dance between the specific and the universal, the personal and the professional, the immediate and the timeless. Because this giant in the field of nursing has retired, I am being mentored into how a professional moves from an executive position to one of wisdom keeper. Much more than any idea or story shared, it is the essence and energy of the woman, the courage and integrity of the woman that has shaped and molded my own potential in these arenas. Because of her modeling the promise of what is to be, my private life, as well as the life shared with others, reflects her sacred path toward wholeness.

To be most helpful, a relationship with the mentor enhances the protégé's performance as well as professional and personal development. This is established when the mentor is familiar with the protégé's personal goals and talents, identifying aspects of the protégé's development where growth can be encouraged. This requires knowing the other from an insider's perspective, as well as candor and clarity in establishing parameters for the mentored experience designed to align mutually held values and purposes. This cocreated foundation is enlarged and enriched as the wisdom keeper and protégé continue a dialogue of honesty around successes and failures on their shared journey. A mentor of superior professional achievement with a diverse range of interests and activities offers the greatest potential for the protégé's learning and development. The mentor's publications, involvement in professional organizations on a local or national level, and focused career history reflect a high standard of professional competence and attest to skill in handling political dynamics. The protégé may examine at what cost the mentor achieved professional success. An analysis of the mentor's value system and priorities will disclose the degree of balance between experiences outside the job sphere and professional activity. The issue of the mentor's sex is an item of debate. The complexities of male and female dynamics are avoided if one selects a mentor of the same sex.

However, the presence of female nurse leaders in top administrative positions is still a rare phenomenon. An opposite sex mentor may expose the protégé to the "masculine" or "feminine" point of view pertaining to professional issues and concerns, leading to a broader human perspective. The most important factor to consider in choosing the mentor is a willingness to give personal time and attention. The mentor can honor the relationship and facilitate the learning experience only by devoting personal energy to it.

MAXIMIZING THE ROLE OF PROTÉGÉ

A journey toward wisdom requires energy. The current reality of nursing leaders' lives is that they are filled with consuming demands in a chaotic, changing world. Leonard (1992) identifies life issues that are energy leaks. Conquering these issues would release energy for the protégés' acquisition of mastery. *Maintaining physical fitness* is an essential beginning. By being in touch with our bodies and nature, we experience healthy living on this planet. *Acknowledge the negative and accentuate the positive*—denial inhibits energy, while realistic acknowledgment of the truth releases it. A positive attitude in dealing with the negative is the key to achievement. *Tell the truth*—lies and secrets are poison, as energy is devoted to deceiving and hiding. Truth-telling includes sharing your own feelings while honoring those of others. *Honor, but don't indulge, your dark side*—suppressing parts of our personality requires energy. *Set priorities*—decide where you will use your potential energy. Liberation comes through accepting limits. By setting priorities you add clarity to life, and clarity creates energy. *Make commitments and take action*—the journey to wisdom is ultimately goal-less; the journey is taken for its own sake. However, intermittent goals help refocus one's path and commitment; and commitment is energy. *Get on the path and stay on it*—over the long haul there is nothing like the path of mastery to lead an energetic life. Disciplined, regular practice not only elicits energy but tames it. The wisdomkeeper's journey is one of perspective, which keeps the flow of energy going during both high and low moments. Energy can't be hoarded; it is not built up by disuse. Unaccompanied by positive action, rest may depress you. Depression, discontent, violence, and crime can be traced to unused energy and untapped potential. Synergy of creative energy is the life-force that can heal the world.

ON BECOMING A WISDOM KEEPER

A goal for the discipline of nursing is to develop wisdom keepers within the profession who will facilitate the emergence of a critical mass of nurse leaders for a re-forming health care system. While obviously benefiting the protégé, the mentor-protégé relationship fulfills personal and professional needs of both. A mentor derives satisfaction in witnessing the protégé advance within the profession. For seasoned wisdom keepers, the protégés' success eases mentors' transitions to retirement as they see someone continuing to advance the contributions they have made during their careers. Having protégés underscores the mentor's own status and power while simultaneously serving the profession. The lack of suitable mentors for up-and-coming nursing professionals, particularly women, is a dangerously limiting condition for the profession as well as for the individual nurse. Bidwell and Brasler (1989) call mentorship the "essence of adulthood" and suggest that it may be impossible to become a mentor without first having had a mentor. Whether the mentor or the protégé makes the first invitation, a conscious commitment to the mentor relationship has enormous potential for mutual enrichment and benefit for the individual and the profession. The individual and collective power and effectiveness of professional nursing will depend on our willingness to support each other on the path to wisdom.

A Leader's Mentors
by Clara L. Adams-Ender

Q: Who have been your most significant mentors during your nursing career?

CAE: Let me first say what nursing means to me, and then we'll discuss mentoring. Nursing is a caring profession. But you must first care about yourself to care for others. In all fields, including nursing, we must teach others to care more about self. Caring is a major need in society. Increasing incidences of personal and group violence are indicators that caring about self and others is missing. Much of what I do with nurses is to impart the importance of mentoring, which is about caring for both self and others. My parents were my first mentors. My nursing philosophy and experiences have been influenced profoundly by two primary and significant nurse mentors.

My first nurse mentor was Brigadier General Lillian Dunlap. She was a lieutenant colonel when I met her, and I was a lieutenant in the Army Nurse Corps Career course. She said to me, "You've got to get your act together. We've got to get you educated." One of the first things that Lil Dunlap pushed me to develop was my philosophy about nursing. She invited and challenged me to develop ideas and thoughts about vital issues facing nursing, questions about where you were in the profession and what you were about, your beliefs about the practice and patients. I found out that I didn't know enough about the issues, but she invited me to read and become educated and deeply involved in the profession. I have passed this challenge on to others. Lil Dunlap told me to come to her with problems. I went to her about a struggle I was having with a classmate. She said, "Your first responsibility is to yourself. If you keep your focus on your work, I will help you get where you want to go." My parents, who were my important early mentors, said "Always obey your elders and listen when they are talking." And so I listened and followed the advice of my mentor, to my eternal gratitude. She also helped me see that self-absorbed or oppressed persons cannot mentor. However, one must address one's self first and then go on to give to others. It changed my career, knowing Lil Dunlap. From 1964 until 1974, she had a direct influence on my career moves. For example, I wanted to be assigned to the Medical Training Center at Fort Sam Houston, Texas, but I was told that I didn't have enough experience. I called Lil and told her they didn't want me. The chief of the Nursing Service Division subsequently gave me this assignment primarily because Lil Dunlap asked her to give me a chance—that I would do a good job. Although we were never assigned together, we talked regularly on the phone or sent notes to each other. Lil watched out for me. After 30 years, this relationship continues to today. She is now retired and lives in San Antonio. She never lost faith in my being an original thinker. I knew well her "fire." She was always soft-spoken, but her knowledge, power, and authority were known by those around her. We share many values. One of the major things I liked about Lil was her no-nonsense, practical approach.

Q: What, in your opinion, is mentoring?

CAE: Mentoring is a special loving relationship between two people. The mentor tells you what you *need* to hear versus what you *want* to hear. Lil's style of mentoring is similar to how I now mentor: encourage independent thinking and be a free spirit. I also make sure that my protégés seek somebody to mentor. One should always take on protégés and learn from them. Also, it is important to know that when someone is looking up to you, you are not always aware how much that person values your opinion. It is important for a mentor to help build confidence as well as share ideas about the profession. This may occur at different stages. The exchange of ideas and mutual learning are important mentoring aspects to be passed from one person to another and from one generation to the next. We also should be kind to each other, a virtue to be valued in a mentor relationship.

Q: Who was your second significant mentor?

CAE: My second great nursing mentor was Colonel Katherine Galloway. I met her in 1974 when I was the assistant vice president of nursing during my first administrative position at Ft. Meade, Maryland, and Katy was the chief nurse. She was a very kind, soft-spoken, and powerful person, like my mother. Katy was a role model of kindness for me. Kindness doesn't always mean that you must be pleasant and agreeable. Sometimes you may need to give someone a swift kick, which Katy could do unflinchingly. Katy was a role model for me as a woman; she portrayed femininity and womanhood at the same time she was able to use power and influence to her advantage and do it well. Katy helped women and nurses gain a lot of high ground. In my position with Katy, I was given the responsibility and freedom to run the daily operations with her support. It was a deep and trusting relationship. Katy died in 1985, and I delivered the eulogy at her funeral.

Q: How does mentoring prepare one for leadership in the profession?

CAE: To get into a leadership position, you have to look to a leader for guidance. The same characteristics are required across the board for leaders: vision, philosophy, relationships, values, knowledge, energy, and endurance (a combination of stamina and persistence). A mentor helps one get organized as a leader, even to aspire to be a general in the army. Traditionally, in the army, women couldn't be generals, even though they might be as good in their skills as generals. I decided that I could be in charge of others, but I realized that I needed more than a bachelor's degree. When I wanted to find out what leaders were about, I looked to the generals. I needed to find out what they knew and what they would do to help others. I asked them, "How did you get where you are today?" They willingly told me and showed me how to best accomplish my goals.

Q: Were these male mentors different from your female mentors?

CAE: I also was encouraged by the male generals. Since I had grown up playing with my brothers and their friends, I was very much at ease with men in the work world. I was in the army for 11 years before there were female generals, so I had to learn from male generals. They taught me a lot about the values and what qualities to develop as a general. I learned to deal with my own dilemmas and the fit or nonfit of my values. When the values were not in the "right" order, I had to sort them out. I had a number of nonnursing leadership mentors, and the preponderance of them were men. They taught me about leadership, how to behave, how to lead, and how to develop other leaders. Male and female mentors teach some of the same things, but they do it in a different order. Men are competitive and often try to knock others down to gain a hierarchical position. I don't think like that. Competition is not a woman's first value—we are community oriented and look at how people are feeling and where they stand. Women tend to pass out kudos to each other, but men don't pass out many to each other. Women write notes and let others know when they have done well. Women are into relationships. Men also like it when they get special attention because they are human beings. They enjoy receiving the kudos, but have more difficulty praising each other.

Q: In a male-dominant organization, what did male mentors give to you?

CAE: They helped me look objectively at the workplace and

deal with problems in a decisive way. My female mentors were also decisive, but felt free to change their minds and "switch it up." I, too, changed my mind if I felt it was necessary. I tried to combine both of these values—making the best decision at the right time and not being too proud to change my mind if indicated. It is necessary to have the courage of your convictions and to be able to confront situations that require confronting. Of course, this may cause conflict, but it is important to get it out on the table, discuss the conflict, and solve the problem.

Q: Would you say that racism in society was ever an obstacle for you as a protégé or mentor?

CAE: I view an obstacle as something to be overcome as opposed to stopping me. One gets through an obstacle—over, under, or around. For me, this view is a positive thing. As an African American, I believe that I have something to offer. If I were not there to offer it, it would not be part of the equation. If I didn't offer, it might not get done. I have strong self-confidence. I have something to give—I need to give without hindrances or prohibitions. There are things I can do nothing about. But I must be this person that I was born to be. We waste a lot of time being the person we are if we are focusing on the person that we aren't, but want to be. I spend a lot of time being the person that I am. I believe that factors such as skin color, religion, ethnicity, and gender don't need to be obstacles if you have a strong sense of self, are persistent, and have mentoring support. I've had a lot of fun.

Mentoring: An Interactive Process

by Ruth Watson Lubic

The process of mentoring, to me at least, is only partly an intellectual exercise. Indeed, the success of the process is as much dependent on the affective relationship developed between mentor and protégé as it is on planned cerebral interchanges. My work in setting up a freestanding birth center to serve low-income families (The Childbearing Center of Morris Heights, Bronx, New York) reinforced me as protégé equally as much as it did me as mentor.

I would like to emphasize the interactive and humbling quality of the mentoring process through recounting an experience in working with minority, inner-city, childbearing women in which I learned a great deal about the strength and beauty of many families living there. I felt very much in the protégé role and was startled when one of the women referred to me as her mentor. It embarrassed me to know that she apparently was oblivious of the great gifts of information and understanding that *she* was providing me. In truth, on one level I was counseling her about my world of health care policy making, but I believe my effect on her paled beside her effect on me. The motherhood experience, as it was provided in the Childbearing Center of Morris Heights, had empowered the women and their families to a degree beyond my most optimistic expectations. They were ready and eager not only to participate in their own health care, but also to initiate positive social change in their communities. I, in turn, was ready and eager to see their experience replicated in every inner city in the country. Parenthetically, I believe that by focusing on the weaker families living in low-income areas rather than emphasizing the stronger ones, we have missed a great opportunity to create change. The strength of these families and their readiness to be involved in social change are illustrated by the following quotation from the mother referred to previously in which she speaks to those who made available the unique care provided at the birth center:

> It's very rare that a person's career choice or purpose in life allows [him or her] the divine opportunity to touch and effect positive change in people's lives the world over. . . . I've had the opportunity to do just that. I have traveled to many states, cities, and little towns on behalf of childbearing women everywhere as a consumer advocate, representing all women's rights to optimum health care and their birthright to birth as they choose! As we all know, the paths we choose directly affect the development (or demise) of our character. Thank you again for the opportunity to develop and expand my character through working with you, learning from you, and growing with you, as we each develop and expand each other's character with our own life's experiences. In one of the greatest racially saturated and divided cities in the world, my greatest accomplishment, for which I will forever remain indebted, is helping to create a woman's place to birth, free of

racial issues and impositions. . . . We are all aware (or should be) of the intense racism imposed on every aspect of non White peoples' lives in this city (and many others). In spite of this, when I walked into the [birth center] to register for pre-natal care, I knew the moment I walked in that I was home. When I saw, came to know, and chose my midwife . . . when I saw Ruth holding the door open for me as I arrived for my son's birth, came to know her, and chose her as one of my mentors, I knew I was in a racism-free environment. For many of you this may seem "not so important," or "tangential to real issues," or not even a real issue at all . . . but to all non White people this is one of the most important aspects of being able to live life in peace. For where there is no justice (and there is none in racism), there is no peace!" (Zakiyyah Madyum, personal communication, August 1995)

Further evidence of the interactive effects of mentoring can be found in the way these women and families became free to express to resident physicians what their experiences in conventional hospital settings had meant to them and how demeaned they had felt. They could have angrily lashed out when given the opportunity to "present" at the backup hospital's family practice rounds. Instead, they "told it like it is" and deeply touched the physicians, speaking with honesty and directness as empowered women—women whose self-esteem had been raised by the simple but magical act of "giving birth" rather than "being delivered." We nurse-midwives mentored them and taught them how to do it. They, in turn, humbled and mentored us with the way they used their success. It was an experience of riches for all of us—families, nurse-midwives, and physicians alike.

Full Circle: Peer Mentorship

by Caroline Erni and Susanne Greenblatt

We still remember our first impressions of each other as we started staff nurse positions in a busy New York City emergency room 14 years ago. Susanne, who had recently left a charge position at another city ER, seemed all-knowing to Caroline; Caroline's adventures as a nurse living out of a tent in Wyoming made her seem wholesome and almost unreal to Susanne. Since we were an orientation group of two, we spent a lot of time together. We could never have predicted that a lifelong personal and professional relationship of peer mentoring had begun.

Susanne: All my ER stories that captivated audiences at parties also worked on Caroline. In the ER, telling stories can be a way of passing on knowledge. Occasionally, you can navigate an unfamiliar situation by recalling a coworker's story. Of course, the amount of stories one has is directly proportional to one's years of experience, so newcomers become listeners and learners simultaneously. At the time, I had no idea that Caroline was learning from my stories.

Caroline: I was immediately impressed with Susanne the first time I met her. She was friendly and self-assured. Her experiences in the ER were unimaginable to me at that point in my career. Susanne's ability to extend herself to me made me so much more comfortable in what could have been an overwhelming experience. I remember feeling exhilarated and terrified simultaneously. I wasn't exactly what you'd consider "street smart." Susanne reassured me continuously—"You'll be fine." It seemed she had more confidence in me than I had in myself. She accepted my errors as part of the learning process and supported me in my anguish over mistakes. More important, she taught me how to do it right for the next time. As my anxiety level began to decrease with new knowledge and skills, I began to look forward to the evenings I would be working with Susanne. She was so willing to give of herself to her patients and to her peers. She was constantly teaching. Beyond that she even taught me that working in a busy ER is something that can be enjoyed and that there is humor in everything, if you stop to take the time to look. Our dinner breaks were spent in the diner across the street where we could view the influx of ambulances and patients. It was in these 60-minute respites that we listened to each other and kept each other sane. We created our own forum for critical incident stress debriefing long before it became an identified need in health care. These sessions could be tearful, humorous, or soul searching in an attempt to find answers to often unanswerable questions. By practicing beside Susanne, I began to see and know the genuine compassion and honesty that has shaped much of my moral and ethical decision making. She taught me to leave aside biased judgment in dealing with the often unorthodox and at times illegal lifestyles of many of our clientele and to listen carefully to find out what their real needs were. As I gained experience, I was able to look beyond the superficial appearances and the stereotypes and accept people for their basic humanity. My time working with Susanne in the emergency room left an indelible mark on me. It has shaped who I have become and how I approach people and life in general.

After a year and a half in the emergency room, Caroline left to work in the NICU [Neonatal Intensive Care Unit]. One year later Susanne decided that she was ready to pursue a different avenue in nursing. As she looked for another nursing position as stimulating and challenging as her ER position had been, Caroline's success stories about the babies in the NICU began to sound appealing. So, the tables turned. Susanne became the NICU novice, guided and mentored by Caroline's knowledge and experience.

Susanne: While we were in the NICU, the exchange of knowledge between us lost any work or friendship boundary. True respect for each other's knowledge helped me become a stronger nurse. For instance, during my first year in the NICU, I began to believe that the nurses who were parents had a different perspective about the patients. This was confirmed when Caroline became pregnant. She and her husband shared with me so many of their thoughts, feelings, and expectations about the baby that I began to appreciate how the bonding process begins before the baby is born. I learned much more than clinical skills from Caroline. The demands of parenting relocated Caroline to her home. Our friendship remained a constant in the continually changing complexity of our lives. There were many long-distance phone calls, sharing problems and successes. When Caroline did finally return to work, it was only to leave. Her inability to separate her personal feelings from the parents of critically ill infants left her immobilized to provide needed support.

Caroline: I remember the evening I knew I had to leave the NICU. I had to do a heel stick glucose on a beautiful 8-pound baby who was on a ventilator and was essentially brain dead as a result of an air embolus. The mother looked at her infant lovingly, and all I could do was cry. I couldn't say a word to comfort her. I thought about my own beautiful child sleeping at home and knew that this mother would never see her child smile at her. Her tragedy might as well have been mine. I resigned within a week. In her usually supportive fashion, Susanne understood my reasons for leaving and empathized. She told me for the thousandth time, "You'll be fine."

Susanne: In a laughable way, I felt that Caroline had abandoned me. First of all, it was fun to work with her. Second, I would now have to ask the other nurses all the questions that I asked Caroline. It was safe to expose my stupidity to her, but I cringed at the thought of asking the other staff nurses at least 50 questions a day. It was indeed a humbling experience to learn to ask for help from people who could possibly judge me as ignorant or inept.

So once again the paths of our careers took different directions. Caroline joined the Emergency Room of a local hospital, while Susanne tried to reach the expert level in the NICU. We worked apart for 5 years, but continued to share thoughts on professional issues. Eventually, we both held management jobs. We fleshed out ideas and strategies on patient care as well as staff developmental issues.

Susanne: I ended up back in the ER, returning as a head nurse. I desperately needed Caroline (who was enjoying time at home after the birth of her second child) on the front line.

Caroline: I remember well the recruitment speech I was given by Susanne. It had been five years since I had worked in the ER where she was now employed. Since then, there had been a multitude of technological advances along with a rapidly increasing patient population and acuity level. Susanne was adamant that it would be like getting back on a bicycle: "Once a good nurse, always a good nurse. Don't you want to fix the problems we've been identifying for years? Now's your chance!" Susanne can be very persuasive. She had ideas of what I could achieve long before I had the time to think about them. I now had a second child, Susanne, named after one of the most honest, moral persons my husband and I have ever known.

Susanne: I needed Caroline in the ER for several reasons. A lack of strong nurses created a twofold problem: the patients were not getting the care they deserved, and there were no staff role models to help bring the nurses to a higher level of practice. Although Caroline might be rusty, I knew that she could quickly readjust to a busy ER. We needed someone who held a similar nursing belief system and who could influence the staff. If we had patience, someone on the management team would eventually leave, opening a spot for Caroline. What a thrill to imagine that we would be in charge of the ER where we had started our careers several years ago. . . . Of course, good managers can always predict the future! A position became available, and Caroline joined the management team. My role changed to include responsibility for education on the unit. We were finally able to try to put into action the philosophy that had been instilled in us many years ago: "THE PATIENT COMES FIRST."

Caroline: It was finally happening. I was the head nurse in a Level 1 trauma center. I couldn't believe it! A lifelong dream had come true. . . . I was ready to change things. The management team was in place. Our goals were realistic. First, the patient, any patient, is treated with respect and dignity. Second, the professional and educational levels of the nurses working in the emergency department had to be elevated. My promotion to manager was a difficult transition. Without the mentorship and support of Susanne and her ability to refocus on goals, I'm not sure I could have made it. Susanne's commitment to education on the unit was already bringing about a change in the delivery of patient care. Hiring was no longer viewed as, "If you want a job, I have an opening." Instead, individuals were screened for genuine enthusiasm and a love of nursing. The "hazing" of nurses as they entered the nursing practice on the unit was not to be tolerated. We had witnessed the downfall of many new nurses to the wrath of a ruthless preceptor. A positive mentoring experience became a unit goal with ongoing support and continuing education.

Susanne and Caroline: There was finally light at the end of the tunnel. After a year and a half, the staff was working in the right direction. Continuing education was in place on the unit, and nurses felt they were being treated fairly and supported strongly. It is hard to describe the feeling of obtaining a long-desired goal. That we had come full circle together was almost unthinkable. That we would continue to mentor and influence each other through our entire careers was certain.

The Privilege and Responsibility of Mentoring

by Hattie Bessent

The need for mentoring is a critical concern for the future of America's nurses. This critical juncture is related to the rapidly

changing parameters of health care systems and the revolution-
ary role changes that nurses are experiencing and will confront
increasingly in the future. Nurses must be educated continuously and nurtured in their roles of caring and comforting
humankind. Mentoring occurs at many levels and should be
continuous, goal directed, and under the aegis of a capable person who has the best interest of the protégé as the focal point.
The mentor's philosophy needs to be a simple but powerful one:
to serve the protégé as a trusted teacher and counselor. In my
role as mentor to many nurses, I have had to participate constantly in the self-examination of my attributes, my protégés'
visions and goals, and visions about what I believed the protégés
could become. This type of examination has brought me full circle in the pursuit of my own strengths and limitations in serving
others. In my self-examination, I have discovered that a mentor
for nurses, especially minority nurses, must be relentless and
possess a clear vision about futuristic possibilities for the protégé. Many nurses have a vision limited to traditional roles in
nursing. My vision for nurses, however, includes both excellence
in the traditional roles and an expansion in paradigm shifts that
uncover other opportunities in health care systems. I believe that
these paradigm shifts place nurses at the pith of caring and comforting, accompanied by a multitude of responsibilities and possibilities. Some protégés have had to be convinced that my
vision for them was possible and attainable. In fact, protégés, on
occasion, would need to be gently guided and directed into an
exploratory process where various scenarios were developed
and critiqued.

The ANA Ethnic/Racial Minority Doctoral Fellowship
Program provided me the unique opportunity to galvanize my
visions for many nurses and then gently persuade them to participate with me in vision exploration. A core component of this
philosophy is related to gently persuading others to have visions
about their possibilities. As their mentor, I frequently provide a
foundation of faith and courage on which their embryonic vision
rested until their own competence and determination emerged.
At times, my faith and courage were tested by my own fleeting
doubts that naturally accompany ambiguities and the unknown.
Nevertheless, the dedication to the mentor role sustained me. The
vivid visions that I perceived and the changing demands of
health care have made me relentless in my mentoring. The

Doctoral Fellowship Program placed me in the presence of many capable minority nurses. At times, the barriers that they confronted in the pursuit of their goals could be as powerful as my desire to gently guide and teach them. Again, the dedication to our work and the desire to be available to them when they needed me created dynamic mentor-protégé relationships. The dedication to work is essential for the survival of the mentor-protégé relationship. To teach, tutor, counsel, and help with unraveling missions requires many hours of critical thought. This work involves the development of networks to assist doctoral students and others in various pursuits. This dedication to work evolved into mentor-protégé sessions for clarity, alternative-seeking strategies, conflict resolution, and the demonstration of the importance of sustaining long-term relationships. Hours dedicated to this mission extended into the early morning and late night. The results have been phenomenal.

The roles and functions of the mentor and protégé must be understood clearly. The negotiations occur overtly and covertly. For example, it was essential that I encourage the protégé to explore the worlds of academia, research, and practice. It was my role, however, to assist the protégé to grow and develop in whatever professional arena he or she had chosen. The professional growth and development of the protégé, at times, involved helping family members to understand the vision of the protégé. This vision could be contrary to the family's vision. In some instances, the protégé's new vision was distinctly different from the visions that family members shared. Talking with family members, explaining new possibilities and opportunities, was a constant challenge. I have had conversations with husbands, fathers, mothers, aunts, uncles, children, and friends. These conversations were at times anxiety provoking, but essential. Together, we sustained a vision. Family and friends became the extended foundation of faith and courage for the protégé, until his or her own competence emerged. The protégé's success was often linked to improved family and community communication, support, and resources. Perhaps one of the most rewarding outcomes was observing family members acquire the desire to mentor the student. When family members support, nurture, and encourage nurses, they share many family and community functions. The protégé is exposed to additional alternatives, and visions are created and maintained. This outcome strengthens family, friendship, and community ties that enhance additional mentoring of minority nurses and many, many others—a generational outcome.

One of my protégés is a brilliant young nurse researcher and clinician, who is the first college graduate in her family. She is nationally known for her commitment to clinical research and excellence in practice, and is employed at a prestigious institution. She has been successful in attaining research funds from the National Institutes of Health and has written several books. In addition, she frequently receives requests to participate in international programs, conduct workshops, and teach. By any standard, she is a successful and dynamic professional. We have reflected on her career and the factors that influenced her to commit to her vision plan. We met when she was a hospital staff nurse. Her vision included being promoted some day to nurse manager on her unit. We talked at national conferences and corresponded by mail and phone. Over a period of about 3 years, we developed her vision plan, constructing goals and a time line. After she received her master's degree, I encouraged her to persevere. About a year later, we had numerous phone conversations about doctoral study. By telephone she introduced me to her husband, and he and I, over time, discussed the possibilities of her studying for a Ph.D. and the positive impact that this accomplishment could have on their entire family. Her mother and aunt also needed to understand the significance of the Ph.D. Within the year, I had developed a telephone relationship with my protégé's family, including her three children, but they still did not understand the nature and significance of the Ph.D. I knew my protégé's vision plan was extremely active when she telephoned me one day and requested that she and her family have lunch with me; they would drive to Washington and meet me at a designated place. I knew that I would need to respond immediately, for visions can be fleeting; however, this one was being cemented. Several weeks later, I met my protégé, her husband, mother, aunt, and three children. We enjoyed our lunch together and talked about future goals. I was aware that all of the adults would have to believe in her vision plan—she would need their cooperation, support, and blessing. By the time we departed, the entire family had agreed to support her, and they expressed gratitude to me for explaining the "Ph.D. thing." Her mother was elated about the notion that her daughter could have "one of those things, too." In the fall of that year, my protégé began her doctoral studies, and 3 years later, she graduated. My protégé recently commented to me, "You know, I am a mentor now . . . and soon I will be able to mentor almost as well as you do!"

Mentoring is a privilege and an awesome responsibility. I have met this responsibility in a relentless and dedicated manner. There also is a deep sense of gratitude that is internalized, as I have had the opportunity to influence the lives of hundreds of nurses and their families.

Mentoring and Nursing's Relational Capacities

by Julie MacDonald

The process of mentoring is akin to a number of the core processes within the essence of nursing. Caring, knowing, accepting, facilitating, and empowering are key capacities needed in nurses for them to be fully with the patient and to see the patient's human health experience through his or her eyes. These capacities in nurses relate to what Lamb and Stempel (1994) refer to as nursing's "insider" role. They are critical in helping patients achieve health, in Nightingale's sense of not only being well "but using well every power that they have" (Dolan, Fitzpatrick & Herrman, 1983, p. 164). These capacities as integral components of nursing's essence and work should make the role of mentor a natural one in nursing's service to patients and to each other. My personal journey throughout my nursing career has been to embrace the privilege that comes with relationships that foster the ability to be truly with another and to build accountability for these relationships, both at the bedside and within the profession. What has been perplexing, frustrating, and an obstacle to growth in nursing has been the lack of development and accountability for the capacities of caring, knowing, accepting, facilitating, and empowering in service to one another.

When I assumed my first nursing management role after 10 years at the bedside, the absence in the work environment of these capacities, necessary for nursing and mentoring, was a glaring need and an opportunity. Luckily, as naive as I was, I was smart enough to know that fostering the necessary capacities was larger than one manager's work, requiring the abilities of every nurse on the unit. What I achieved during my 1st year and a half in that role was the trial of a framework that affected both the capacities within nurses, the practice of nurses, and the social environment in which we worked. Moreover, the framework provided the basis for the future transformation of nursing leadership in my subsequent role.

Carl Rogers's (1961) work in client-centered therapy served as a leadership template for me, as it had in my clinical practice. Quickly I could see the relevance of Rogers's theory to any situation in which development of the person and release of the individual's capacity was the goal. I not only applied this model in my work as nurse, manager, mentor, and colleague, but perhaps, most important, I began to utilize it in developing others in their capacity to mentor. Rogers's foundation for the growth-promoting climate involves three conditions. The first condition is *genuineness, realness*, and *congruence*. It calls for mentors to be themselves without any professional fronts or personal facades. Being ego-fit is critical for the mentor in this first condition, and the transparency of self is required. Being genuine results in a maximum space for both the mentor and the person being mentored to be and ultimately to become. The second condition in creating a climate for change and development is that of *acceptance, caring*, or *unconditional positive regard* for wherever the person being mentored is on the journey and in his or her learning. Rogers describes this as a "non-possessive caring" (1978, p. 10). There is no judgment or evaluation involved. This attitude provides a nurturant atmosphere but not an all-knowing, forcing one. It requires a thorough self-acceptance on the part of the mentor to be able to offer unconditional regard to the protégé. The third condition and facilitative aspect of this relationship is *empathetic understanding*. Empathy is described as sensing accurately the personal meanings and feelings that are being expressed by the one being mentored (Rogers, 1978). The mentor also must be able to communicate this understanding. This reflection often helps one gain a new depth in understanding the significance of this meaning to learning and development. Of the three conditions, this one is often the easiest, for it can be learned as a skill and an attitude. Moreover, it is an integral part of every nurse's work with patients.

It is the first two conditions, however, that I have come to recognize could be my life work with nurses in advancing a learning, developing, and mentoring environment. This is where my story begins. I assumed the vice presidency for nursing in the same organization less than 2 years into my first management position. My goal was to develop a nursing leadership team that embraced Rogers's three conditions of *genuineness, acceptance,* and *empathetic understanding* in their relationships with each other and ultimately in their work with their staffs. The first few years were focused on skill development in the nursing management accountabilities. At that time the nurse-manager role had a new identity, and like the socialization of all nurses, this group of managers first had to get the technical, task-focused aspects of their role down pat. Soon after, structure and space were created to begin the mentoring process and to change the cultural and social environment throughout the nursing department to one that recognized and supported the potential in each member. The work occurred at multiple levels within the department. Most directly, I targeted my efforts with a group of 5 directors, who in turn targeted their efforts with 20 nurse managers, who in turn targeted their efforts with over 600 staff nurses. Systems were developed to support the movement within the nursing department. Perhaps most profound and far-reaching was the building of nursing leadership standards that incorporated these capacities and the subsequent development of a peer-review system for every member of the leadership team.

There are many anecdotes that describe what happened in the process of peer review utilized with the group of nursing leaders. The process became as instrumental in the transformation of individuals as did the standards and expectations themselves. At the same time, the peer-review process became one more vehicle for bringing Rogers's relational conditions alive. This learning and change happened over a number of years. For some it was far easier than others, because of where they were in their own personal journeys of trust of self and with others. In addition, embracing these conditions in relation to one another called for a genuine willingness to let go of some of the "victim" behaviors many nurses have adopted. A substantial amount of open reflection about this process and the resultant individual and collective effect occurred both formally and informally. The investment by individuals had a mutual benefit for all involved, for one cannot create this type of relationship that facilitates growth in others without measurably growing oneself. For this reason, and because of the number of persons involved, this not only resulted in the growth and development of many individuals, but had an enormous influence on the work and practice environment. The trickle down and up effect of this effort is palpable and was notably recognized as the dissertation focus by an affiliated nursing professor at a local university. Stejskal (1992) states, "Nurses at a midwest hospital thrive in a person-centered community that values the contributions of each unique individual. Nurses are supported in their creative endeavors with the power, freedom and space to serve the patient and the institution" (p. 236).

As I reflect on the developmental mentoring accomplishments by nursing leadership, I also would include mutuality, affiliation, a deep emphasis on human relations and the potential of each individual, greater acceptance and valuing of intuition and feelings, and widespread empowerment at every level within the department. Moreover, the standards once embraced at the nursing leadership level have been incorporated into the clinical ladder for staff nurses and into the leadership competencies for all management roles across the entire health system. The focus on developmental relationships among nurses and within nursing that are based on *genuineness, acceptance,* and *empathetic understanding* can have a profound effect on individual development toward full potential and on the social practice environment. My personal bias is that the earlier in one's career this mentorship occurs, the better. The notion of incorporating aspects of this framework into nursing education might be our greatest hope for developing this capacity and accountability toward one another. It is my belief, however, that it is not responsible or appropriate to stand by and wait for tomorrow's generation of nurses. The pathway to today's nurse can be found by a recommitment to nursing's essence and applying these processes to our work with each other. Not only will we find greater individual wholeness and growth, but a new appreciation for the potential of nursing's collective wholeness.

Mentoring Behaviors versus Mentoring Relationship: A Dissenter's Perspective

by Sandra K. Hanneman

I support the classical definition of mentoring as a long-term, developmental relationship, and disagree with attempts to define it simply as discrete, albeit desired, behaviors. This developmental relationship is founded in tradition and needs to be reemphasized as a vital part of our profession. The 10-year developmental relationship between Athena and Odysseus and his son in *The Odyssey* serves as the source of the mentoring concept. It is not Athena's discrete behaviors but the cumulative effect of the behaviors that resulted in Odysseus's growth and success. Levinson, Darrow, Klein, Levinson, and McKee (1978) emphasized this notion of time in a seminal work on adult male development, finding that the mentor relationship lasts 2 to 3 years on the average and can last from 8 to 10 years. Thus one attribute of mentorship is that the relationship endures over time, encompassing— but surely not defined by—discrete behaviors. The shared vision of mentor and protégé for the protégé's eventual success guides a mentoring relationship. It is precisely the promise that both persons see in the protégé that serves as the basis of the relationship. This promise justifies the investment of time and energy needed to sustain the relationship over several years.

I believe two persons enter into a mentoring relationship only when there is differential status. The protégé believes that the mentor has achieved success and has characteristics that the protégé wishes to possess or emulate. Such characteristics include the power of the mentor to open doors for the protégé— power steeped in and derived from the mentor's accomplishments. The notion of equal status, as in peer-peer mentoring, is an oxymoron. One of the persons in the relationship must have survived the perils of career advancement to advise, coach, and teach the other. Without differential status, we are talking about support, sharing experiences, or some phenomenon other than mentoring. Indeed, protégé achievement of equal status with the mentor signals the end of the mentoring relationship (Levinson et al., 1978). Philosophical fit (i.e., the "right chemistry") is another attribute of mentoring. We voluntarily associate with, respect, and admire others with whom we feel comfortable. Because mentorship requires time and work, it cannot be mandated, but must be based on free choice. Neither can we mandate admiration, respect, and trust. Thus the idea of assigning mentors is incompatible with the concept of mentoring. Although Odysseus did assign Mentor to protect his son, it was Athena who volunteered to serve Odysseus and his son as guide, adviser, counselor, and protector. Mentoring cannot occur unless both individuals seek the relationship with each other.

Considering the classic literature and research studies, a mental image of mentoring emerges. The image includes: (a) the mentor, (b) the protégé, and (c) the interaction between the mentor and the protégé—the mentor relationship. In keeping with this image, I define the mentor as "a person identified as such by self and the protégé based on achievement of our visions, belief in the protégé's abilities, shared vision for the protégé's accomplishments, and willingness to actively work for the protégé's development." I define the protégé as "a person identified as such by self and the mentor, who admires, trusts, and respects the mentor and the mentor's visions; has visions for self-accomplishment; and lacks consistent and full confidence in own abilities." I define the mentor relationship as "a developmental process that is guided by shared visions of what the protégé can become, promotes personal and professional development of the protégé, and evolves from differential status to peer status."

Every relationship requires at least two persons and is an interactional process. The mentor relationship has the additional requirement of being a developmental process. The primary goal of the mentor relationship is the personal and professional development of the protégé. The characteristics of the mentor (own achievements, belief in the protégé, shared vision, and willingness to invest time and energy) and the protégé (admires mentor's achievements, has own visions, and lacks confidence) are antecedents of the mentoring process. In other words, if the characteristics are not present, whatever process is occurring, it is not that of true mentoring. Concepts such as adviser, teacher, counselor, role model, and preceptor are subsumed within the construct of mentor. Individually and collectively, however, they are far too limited to represent the image of mentor. These concepts are most strongly differentiated from mentoring in terms of vision. The persons assuming such roles may have their visions but are not obligated to concern themselves with the protégé's vision. In each of these roles, the interaction may tilt heavily toward the more experienced person doing active work; the less experienced person may be passive without changing the nature of the role. In contrast, the role of mentor concludes when the protégé's vision is no longer the guiding force.

Herein is the crux of my concern with the reconceptualization of mentoring in nursing. When we reduce mentoring to behaviors, the result is a lack of clarity of the concept. This leads to questionable internal validity of mentoring research and to misconceptions about the prevalence and real value of mentoring in nursing. Research on mentoring in nursing has produced mixed outcomes (Vance & Olson, 1991). I think that failure to consistently demonstrate positive outcomes from mentoring relationships is due to confusion about the concept. Regrettably, absence of consensus about what mentoring is may result in disillusionment with mentoring as a strategy for developing nursing leaders. Vance and Olson think that mentoring is much more pervasive in nursing than I do, that it occurs in all work settings and at all levels of educational preparation. My research (Goodnough-Hanneman, Bines, & Sajtar, 1993; Hanneman, 1996) and that of others (Pyles & Stern, 1983) have demonstrated the beneficial influence of expert nurses on the practice development of nonexpert nurses. However, attributing staff development to mentoring is an invalid inference. We need to recognize the existence of multiple strategies for career development. Although mentoring is surely a career development strategy, not all career development strategies are mentoring.

The complex aspects of mentoring cause empirical measurement dilemmas for researchers. This is not surprising, given that defining the phenomenon is the first rule of measurement. Researchers who confuse multiple concepts are unlikely to advance understanding of any one of them. In their review of mentoring research in nursing, Vance and Olson (1991) confirmed mentoring as process oriented, developmental, and longitudinal. I agree with these essential characteristics, but submit that they are insufficient to differentiate mentoring from other concepts. They also noted that there is widespread development of mentoring programs and that evaluation of such programs may yield nonclassic definitions and new forms of mentoring systems. The words "programs and systems" conjure up a mental image of conformity and institutional focus, whereas classic mentoring suggests a highly personal and individual relationship that transcends institutional affiliation. The idea of mentoring programs or mentoring systems implies assigned relationships, peer status, and disregard for philosophical fit. This is reminiscent of hospital preceptor programs that are designed to socialize new nurses into the traditions, rules, and practices of the setting. These objectives are very different from professional development of new nurses and the achievement of their visions.

Can mentoring behaviors alone produce the desired outcomes? I think not. The classic concept of mentoring has been around a very long time and has been accepted by many disciplines. If the desired outcomes are nursing leaders who achieve wisdom and power, and who, in turn, become wise and trusted leaders for others, discrete behaviors are unlikely to yield noticeable benefits. A sustained commitment to the mentor relationship is requisite to growth of the protégé, which will be achieved by mentoring only if the antecedents exist. A clear understanding of mentoring will enhance our need to nurture nurses in their various practice roles. We have an obligation to each other and to society to ensure that nurses practice with more than a minimum level of competence. There are many strategies to meet this obligation. We should not, however, confuse these strategies with mentoring. Mentoring is a special relationship that requires a substantial investment of time and energy. When we equate lesser investments with mentoring, we diminish the value of mentoring and erroneously convey more widespread use of the concept than reality merits. Role models, teachers, advisers, counselors, and preceptors are distinct from the classically defined mentor. We need to evaluate the contributions of each to the development of nursing, but we should do so with clear conceptual definitions. Blurred images neither advance our knowledge nor contribute to our professional development. Nursing may need new developmental models, but these models will succeed only if they are based on clear understanding and precise definitions.

PART III

The Process of Mentorship

5

Negotiating the Mentor Relationship

Those having torches will pass them on to others (Plato, The Republic).

Mentoring always occurs in relationship. The mentor relationship is a unique human relationship characterized by the reciprocal development of each person. Thus it is beneficial and growth producing for both persons. To succeed, the relationship must be built on a solid foundation of mutual trust, respect, commitment, and shared values. As with any relationship, constant change and evolving occur. Careful communication is essential, as well as ongoing cultivation of the relationship. The two people in the relationship identify with each other through their shared commitments, passions, and concerns. A closeness and emotional attachment to each other frequently develop.

INFORMAL AND FORMAL MENTOR RELATIONSHIPS

Mentors see the unique promise and potential of the protégé. The mentor's gifts are belief in the protégé, encouragement, guidance, and creation of opportunities. Protégés possess the desire to grow and look to people they admire for advice and assistance. Mentoring is bridging into the future—it is transformative, change oriented, and dynamic. Mentoring never rests on acceptance of the status quo and business as usual. Potential, dreams, and expectations are the currency of mentorship. How are these relationships established? There are two varieties of mentor relationships: (a) *informal* or *unplanned* and (b) *formal* or *planned*. Anecdotal and research reports suggest that more and more people are engaging in both forms of these relationships.

Informal mentoring consists of the traditional expert-to-novice relationship and the new, evolving mentorship that includes peer mentoring. Informal mentoring usually occurs when two people are drawn together through "chemistry," mutual attraction, shared interests, concerns, and commitments, and a desire to help and be helped. These relationships frequently develop through work and educational connections, such as superior-to-subordinate or peer-to-peer, the teacher-student relationship, or a preceptored clinical experience. Professional organizations and networks and alumni, work, and community groups also are a source of mentors. Friendships should also not be underestimated for their influence on mentorship. Friends often assume mentoring functions for each other. Out of mutual affection and concern for one another, friends offer advice, lend support, and share connections—all mentoring activities. Sometimes, what started out as a traditional mentor relationship evolves into a friendship. This frequently happens in long-term mentorships. One nursing leader who has had a 40-year relationship with her mentor says that they still meet for dinner, share social events, and that her mentor is called "aunt" by her children, now grown. The following account by a clinical administrative leader illustrates some of the dynamics of informal mentoring.

The "Unintentional" Mentor

by Mary A. Cooke

One of my colleagues said that I became her "unintentional mentor" since it was not a planned "event." It has become evident that mutual respect, common interest and goals, and a desire to grow professionally drew us together. In my case, mentorship has implied colleagueship rather than being a teacher or supervisor. It also explicitly includes friendship, which would not usually be attributed to a purely supervisory relationship. It is now clear to me that this is why I developed a mentoring relationship with two particular nurses over the past 20 years. Propelled by a master's degree into a supervisory role in my 20s, I felt very uncomfortable telling others what to do. Whenever possible, I supervised by role modeling, mentoring, and assisting staff with their work. In this way, I got the satisfaction of doing what I enjoyed and also watching others grow in their skill development and self-confidence. This style of being a mentor-supervisor has been very rewarding and also has drawn talented nurses to work with me. My protégés have also taught me many things about nursing. Because of the mutuality of our interests and goals, it was natural that we would discuss problems and solutions. Although our personalities and even cultural backgrounds are different, there is admiration for each other's strengths, which developed into friendship over time, and has brought us even closer.

I must confess that I never sought the role of mentor; in fact, I didn't really understand what it meant to be a mentor. But I've always been interested in teaching and helping colleagues to increase their knowledge and skills. My goal is to provide the highest quality of care to patients and families. Nurses who share that goal and want to learn have been drawn into a mentoring relationship with me. For me, it has been challenging and gratifying to work with bright, independent nurses who want to learn and grow; this stimulates me to also constantly learn. My mentor relationships were not planned but evolved over time—and I benefited at least equally from these.

Formal or planned is the second type of mentor relationship. This is essentially an organizational application of a traditional person-to-person phenomenon. Formal mentoring occurs in educational and work settings and in professional associations. This is becoming more and more common as an effective way to socialize neophyte students and workers and to provide ongoing development and support for students, employees, and association members. A major issue facing all organizations and professions is preparation for leadership succession, and mentoring is a means to ensure this succession (Drucker, 1988; Holloran, 1993). Many organizations are establishing structures that incorporate the concepts of mentoring into their everyday value systems and working relationships. It is understood that mentoring and learning are intertwined. In "learning organizations," mentors and protégés continually expand their capacity to grow and learn at each stage of their development. In contrast to authoritarian approaches, mentoring programs mitigate the structural, social, and cultural barriers to a sense of community and shared participation.

Mentor relationships throughout an organization or school strengthen creativity and commitment—all so critical in today's chaotic, change-driven world.

Formal work-based programs may exist as a way to anchor new recruits into the organizational culture or as a method to develop long-standing employees (Zey, 1984). Although measuring success of corporate formal mentor programs is difficult, several success indicators continue to be documented: greater commitment to the organization, recruitment improvement, retention and turnover reduction, leadership development, and managerial and leadership succession (Zey, 1997). Organizational mentoring conveys to employees that they are valued and cared about. A mentored employee has a sense of belonging that strengthens his or her commitment to the organization. One organizational expert points out that after formal education is finished, the challenge for creating environments conducive to learning and leadership and career development shifts to employers. He believes that managers, supervisors, and bosses are in the best positions to be mentors and role models (Kotter, 1985). Many organizational theorists believe that one of the most potent shapers of behavior in organizations and in life is *meaning*. Not only leaders, but mentors in an organization, can help us to create meaning and purpose, even in the midst of chaos, uncertainty, and confusion. Mentors can give voice and form to our search for meaning and help us make our work purposeful (Wheatley, 1994).

Various types of school-based programs also are growing in popularity. These programs link student-protégés with mentors who may be peers, more advanced students, teachers, alumni, and practicing professionals. In planned mentoring, potential mentors and protégés are matched with respect to commonalities of goals, interests, and needs. Careful planning, orientation, and training of both mentor and protégé, as well as sustained facilitation, support, and follow-up, are necessary for the success of these programs. Institutionalizing mentor programs is labor intensive and not inexpensive. Formalizing these programs, however, gives mentoring visibility, importance and durability and also creates increased productivity, communication, and motivation (Duff & Cohen, 1993; Murray & Owen, 1991).

Professional associations also are including mentoring as a member service. The mission of the National Association of Women in Education is to address issues in higher education pertaining to the scholarship, leadership development, and advancement of women educators and students. Many of its state chapters are establishing mentor programs. One of these, the North Carolina Association for Women in Education, believes that its mentor program is fast becoming one of the most important association member services. The program provides access to mentors and role models, guidance, support, and coaching, opens the path to productive networks, and expands the learning process and career opportunities (Lee, 1997). In the nursing profession, Sigma Theta Tau International engages members in mentoring activities through a variety of programs at the individual, chapter, regional, and international levels. This international nursing honor society has had mentoring programs for more than 20 years, with leadership advancement as its central purpose. A Chapter-to-Chapter Mentor Program, Regional Coordinating Committee Members for Mentoring, and the Leadership Extern Program are vehicles for both individual and collective mentoring. Rita Gallagher and Doris Edwards state that

> the impact of mentorship within Sigma Theta Tau International has been significant. Chapters and individual members have acknowledged many benefits. Collegial relationships have been enhanced. Vitality, pride, innovation, heightened quality, information sharing, self-evaluation, and renewal give evidence to the value of mentorship in the association. Kanter (1990) observed that America's businesses will be strengthened "when giants learn to dance." By this she means that major corporations must put aside some of the trappings of their competitive cultures and learn to "dance" cooperatively with those organizations with whom they share interests. There are lessons here for nursing and for health care. The isolationist, competitive stance of the past must evolve toward new models of cooperation and collaboration. Lessons learned through mentor relationships are now part of the knowledge and skills base of many nursing leaders. Ongoing, intentional mentoring of nursing's future leaders through a variety of individual and organizational approaches will continue to transform health care. The ability of Sigma Theta Tau International to facilitate scholarship and to foster leadership in nursing through organizational mentoring is a critical international resource for nurses, for the profession, and for our public.

The power of mentorship throughout an entire organization is seen in the following story from one of the three magnet hospitals in the United States.

Mentorship in a Magnet Nursing Department

by Toni Fiore and Laura Cima

In February 1995, Hackensack University Medical Center in New Jersey was awarded the highest recognition of excellence in patient care, the Magnet Hospital Award, sponsored by the American Nurses Credentialing Center. This award reflected 10 years of effort to create an environment in which excellence in patient care is the norm. The Department of Patient Care was the driving force behind the preparation of the hospital for this accomplishment. One initiative critical to our success story is mentorship. Indeed, so important is the concept of mentoring that the American Nurses Association has made this one of the criteria for the Magnet Award. The concept of mentorship is inherent in the philosophy and objectives of the nursing department and in the values of the nursing leadership. Mentoring in our organization occurs at all levels throughout the organization, assumes many forms, is carried out informally and formally, and is internal and external to the organization through our affiliations with numerous educational programs and schools.

A core value in the philosophy of the nursing department is that we must not only take care of our patients but the caregivers as well. Mentorship is the umbrella for caring for the caregiver. Through internal assessment and research studies, we track the presence of mentoring through all recruitment and retention activities—for students, novice and experienced nurses, and nursing leaders. Modes of mentorship are manifested in the student nurse extern program, "lunch with management" (involving executives and staff), student nurse and novice nurse mentor programs, staff committee structures, mentoring partnerships between hospital and educational institutions, and support in role change. One of the cornerstones to the success of the department has been the mentorship of nurses through courses of higher education, advancement to higher positions, career and leadership development, and promotion of advanced practice clinical nursing. We have learned that mentoring is truly a reciprocal process. If staff and leaders are provided the time and tools to mentor one another, they will be successful in giving to and learning from each other and bringing our profession and our organizations into the future.

BEING A MENTOR—FINDING A MENTOR

Regardless of where we are in our personal or professional development, we can all benefit from the mentor connection. Learning and growing are lifelong processes; therefore, we are always in need of people who are willing to be involved with us as we develop. Since there are always people ahead of us and behind us, we can serve as both mentor and protégé. Regardless of the career path we choose, we all have the same need for exploring goals and dreams, finding meaning and purpose in our work, sharing ideas, learning, and understanding the work environment.

How does one become a mentor? Most important, this is dependent on one's attitude. Being willing to serve as a mentor is the first step. This means being on the lookout for promising persons who could benefit from your knowledge, experience, connections, and influence. The next step is reaching out actively and initiating the relationship with the potential protégé. Being involved in another human being's development—whether it be a child, student, peer, protégé, or friend—requires a substantial investment of energy, time, and thought. This investment is both an awesome responsibility and a privilege.

To be a protégé also requires an attitude of willingness—to receive help. Assess your needs and goals and ask for assistance from persons whom you admire and trust. Seek opportunities for networking and meeting other professionals. The workplace and educational settings are venues for finding mentors, as well as professional societies, specialty groups, and alumni associations. Reach out to potential mentors, including both leaders and colleagues, over the course of your career. A requirement for attracting mentors is being dedicated to one's career. A passion for learning and growing makes one an attractive potential protégé. Marketing oneself—assets and strengths—to prospective mentors also is imperative. For those people still outside potential mentoring circles (frequently women and minorities), several strategies are recommended: (a) seek a series of short-term partners who can coach on specific skills; (b) build a board of mentors, a type of advisory panel of experts that changes as needs change; and (c) seek peers and other diverse mentoring partners (Lancaster, 1997).

MAINTAINING THE RELATIONSHIP

The mentor relationship requires the same cultivation and care as any other human relationship. There must be mutual trust and regard and a commitment to each other. In formal, assigned relationships, respect is as essential as liking the person. Usually, some degree of "chemistry" is helpful in giving the relationship spark. In any case, communication is the fuel that will keep mentors and protégés together. Talking, listening, encouraging, challenging one another, and enjoying each other's company—all of these are part of the essence of a vital mentor relationship.

What essential qualities should a mentor and a protégé possess for the relationship to flourish? A good mentor should have the following attributes:

- *Generosity of spirit.* Mentoring is a gift, and requires unselfish givers.
- *Self-confidence and liking of one's self.* Mentors cannot be self-absorbed, oppressed, and unhappy with themselves.
- *Competency.* Possessing security and satisfaction in one's professional life allows one to give to others.
- *Openness to mutuality.* This entails respect for the "other" and a willingness to engage in lifelong learning and growth.

A protégé should possess the following characteristics:

- *Openness to receiving help, learning, and sharing.* This entails not being afraid to ask for advice and guidance.
- *Career commitment and competence.* Motivation and passion for one's work and the profession are essential.
- *Strong self-identity.* This must be maintained in the midst of identification with and imitation of the mentor.
- *Initiative.* One should not wait to be noticed, but make oneself known to potential mentors.

Both mentor and protégé give gifts to each other, and both benefit by this mutual giving. A healthy mentor relationship implies deepening respect, mutual affirmation, and growing collegiality and friendship. Mentoring also is a generational phenomenon, as those who are mentored learn to mentor and pass the gift of mentoring on to future generations of protégés. Rothlyn Zahourek describes it this way:

> For me, being mentored has created opportunities for personal and professional advancement that would not have happened otherwise. For a young adult professional, it was like having ideal parents whom one did not have to resist but from whom one could accept advice and guidance. My mentors' absolute faith in me that I could do a particular job or undertake an area of study was especially helpful. They gave me concrete ideas and worked on projects conjointly with me. They introduced me to others who could help and stimulate; they suggested that I serve on committees or that I join groups relevant to my interests. Occasionally, I was encouraged to start groups that would meet not only my own but my colleagues' interests. These relationships not only enhanced professional success but also were caring and nurturing of self-esteem and self-confidence. As a result, I now mentor others as I have been mentored. My protégés include students, new graduates, and colleagues. These relationships have been satisfying and worthwhile for me and hopefully for them. I have experienced mentoring as generational and trust that my mentoring will encourage others to also mentor.

TROUBLESHOOTING THE MENTOR RELATIONSHIP

No relationship, even one that is developmental and supportive, is perfect. Indeed, there are a few hazards that potentially lurk in mentor relationships. Although the benefits far outweigh these potential dangers, being aware of them can help in avoiding, repairing, or ending problematic situations. The hazards include (a) *unrealistic expectations*, (b) *misuse of power and control*, (c) *competitiveness*, (d) *cloning*, (e) *dependence, and* (f) *overreliance on one person*.

Unrealistic expectations may create difficulties in mentoring. We can expect too little, too much, or the inappropriate. As a result, disappointment, anger, and a sense of betrayal may occur. It is important to be knowledgeable about the mentoring process, its benefits, and limitations. Mentoring is not a panacea for every need or challenge. We must be realistic about the contributions that we can give and receive as mentors and protégés.

Some mentor relationships are characterized by *power and control,* rather than by an empowering and freeing of each other's potential. Some mentors manipulate and exploit their protégés because of their own insecurity. Sometimes they are threatened by the growing strength and independence of the protégé and the possibility of being surpassed in ability and knowledge. They begin to demand excessive loyalty and conformity in the relationship.

Another potential danger is *competitiveness.* Although some degree of competition among colleagues is healthy and normal, excessive competitiveness precludes honesty, trust, and generous sharing. This, in turn, does not allow the full benefits of joining forces through collaboration.

Cloning refers to creating "disciples" who "bow and scrape" and kowtow to every whim of the mentor. This is a severe impediment to the potentiation of the uniqueness of each person in the relationship. Each mentor and each protégé should fulfill their unique potential— become more fully who they can be—not carbon copies of anyone else. Imitation and modeling are positive ingredients of mentoring, but not to the exclusion of the development of one's unique qualities and talents.

Another hazard is *dependence.* Good mentors encourage risk taking, knowing that taking risks and making mistakes are important life activities. Protégés should be encouraged to make their own decisions, with guidance and encouragement from the mentor. This fosters self-confidence and courage. Promoting dependence in mentor relationships stems from the mentor's insecurity and fear of not being needed or being passed by.

An *overreliance on one mentor* also should be avoided. Although traditional mentoring frequently entailed this scenario, having multiple mentors throughout the life-career cycle is the most healthy and desirable situation. Having different mentors for the "different seasons" of one's career provides invaluable perspectives and experiences from a variety of vantage points. In the different life-career journeys that we traverse, it is from a rich diversity of influences that we most benefit.

CONCLUSION

The mentor relationship is akin to other relationships that are driven by mutual affection, love, and sharing. Lucky indeed are the persons who are in these relationships. Mentoring among students, colleagues, and friends adds zest, challenge, joy, and growth to life's experiences. Mentoring gives meaning and direction to one's personal and professional life. Mentor relationships contain healing properties that promote the wholeness and the uniqueness of each person.

PART IV

Contexts for Mentoring

6

Mentoring in the Academic Setting

Imagine classrooms and clinical sites filled with mentor-teachers, who having experienced the value of mentoring, now teach in a framework of affirmation and nurturance of their students in an atmosphere of hope and inspiration (Vance, 1996).

The academic milieu is a prime site for mentorship. Teaching, learning, and mentoring are concerned with the promotion of human development and are therefore closely interrelated. It is widely acknowledged that many teachers assume mentoring functions and also become long-term mentors for their students. Indeed, it has been suggested that as the workplace becomes less stable, with fewer opportunities for the establishment of mentor relationships, the challenge of mentoring new graduates may need to be assumed on an ongoing basis by schools and colleges as well as by specialty groups and nursing associations (Joel, 1997). Students at every stage of their educational experiences, including the rite of passage to the workplace, need not only theoretical and clinical instruction but the wise counsel, nurturing, and guidance of caring mentors. "For more than any other factor, it is the partnership of teacher and student that finally determines the value of an education. In the nurture of that partnership lies the mentor's art" (Daloz, 1986, p. 244). Teachers, too, benefit from mentor connections. Mentoring junior faculty for teaching and scholarship as well as senior faculty for leadership roles can transform the academic environment (Luna & Cullen, 1995). The long-term success and satisfaction of academic executives also has been linked to the mentor connection.

THE UNDERGRADUATE STUDENT

At the 1996 convention of the National Student Nurses Association, the student delegates passed a resolution in "support of the promotion, awareness and development of mentorship programs" (NSNA, 1996). This resolution urged the establishment of mentor programs in schools and nursing organizations and the dissemination of information about the mentor concept. Through this collective action, nursing students have communicated their understanding of the value of mentoring, as well as their desire for this activity in their educational experiences. Mentors for students can be their teachers, clinical-based nurses, senior-level peers, and alumni nurses.

The teacher as intellectual guide and sociocultural role model has been emphasized. Undergraduate nursing students in several studies have reported that mentoring experiences with teachers and clinical nurses improved their communication, technical, organizational, and leadership skills (Atkins & Williams, 1995; Baldwin & Wold, 1993a; Cahill & Kelly, 1989; Clayton, Broome, & Ellis, 1989; Daly & Jones, 1988; Dimino, 1986; Gresley, 1986; Martin, Tolleson, Lakey, & Moeller, 1995; Ramsey, Thompson, & Brathwaite, 1994; Sealy, 1987; Turton & Herriot, 1989). Through active mentoring, students gained self-confidence and felt "cared about" as they progressed toward their educational and professional goals. Their mentors served as important role models and assisted in their career planning. A study of 3rd-year nursing students found that mentorship was particularly important in the early stages of their education. Mentors performed a socializing role as they passed on norms of behavior and nursing routines (Barnshaw, 1995). The reciprocal benefits of teacher-student mentoring are illustrated in these studies because the teacher-mentors believed that their teaching skills had been refined and that their own learning, professional, and personal development was stimulated through mentor partnerships with students. The impact of involved and caring mentors on students' motivation, success, and leadership development is illustrated in the following story.

Mentoring a Student—Growing a Leader

by Cynthia J. Rich Schmus

People achieve great things when they are motivated. This truth alludes to the essence of being mentored as a student. The most powerful aspect of my development as a student was my mentoring relationships. Their effect on my motivation began the day I entered nursing school. From the beginning, I was encouraged by mentor-teachers who saw my potential. I became a leader because people believed in me. If it were not for the faculty who deeply cared about nursing's future and other nurses who sparked my personal vigor, I would not have struggled to make an impact as a student leader.

As a 1st-year student in nursing school at Villanova University, I attended the convention of the Student Nurses Association of Pennsylvania. A confident student leader took her place at the podium of the House of Delegates and led the students through a stimulating process of debating resolutions and discussing issues affecting nursing students. I was invigorated. Someone had obviously seen her potential and pointed her in the right direction. I whispered to our faculty adviser, Dr. Judith Erickson, "I think I would like to be up there one day." Throughout the next year, that faculty adviser became my first mentor. She believed in students and empowered us to lead. At the next state convention, she asked me if a student could nominate me for president so that I could be at that podium! She saw an opportunity for me and encouraged me to reach for it. I took that opportunity, ran for office that year, and won. That single event opened many doors for me over the years. Eventually, I was elected president of the National Student Nurses Association. A strong professional link to an incredible network of nurse leaders is provided by the National Student Nurses Association. Dr. Robert Piemonte, former executive director of the association, mentored me as a student leader. It was as if someone took my hand, showed me the possibilities, then allowed me to lead as one struggling to blossom into a professional. Many nurse leaders, like Dr. Piemonte, essentially mentor the entire nursing profession. They set an example of professionalism, motivate each student to strive for the best that nursing has to offer, and encourage students to offer the best of themselves to nursing. These leader-mentors invest energy in students like myself, thus investing in the future of the profession.

Early in my undergraduate life, I decided that my education would be ongoing. I looked once again to my mentors for their insight about what I needed to seek in graduate study. They provided guidance, support, and learning opportunities, and also challenged me to assess myself. These mentors became part of the path to my choices regarding education, leadership, and networking. Upon graduation, because of my socialization and the foundation that had been laid in my student years, I continued to investigate leadership opportunities both on the job and in professional organizations. Recently, I was elected president of the Alpha Nu Chapter of Sigma Theta Tau International. Last year I was given an award for Excellence in Clinical Practice. Who do you think nominated me for the award? My faculty adviser from my undergraduate program, of course! Here was Dr. Erickson, after all this time, still pointing me in the right direction.

For me, the essence of my professional being was planted the day I entered nursing school. It was nurtured, nourished, and watered by the wisdom of mentors. As a student, developing leadership is a continuous process of learning and being motivated. We need mentors to help us learn these lessons. All of the opportunities that came my way enabled me to take control of my future and to choose exciting paths in nursing. As I was being motivated, I felt a desire to motivate others. Therefore, the powerful circle of mentoring continues. It was through my mentor relationships that I, too, learned to mentor others. To mentor a student is to mold the direction of our profession.

Teaching and learning always occur in relationship. Of particular relevance to nursing, where students are predominantly female, is the research that demonstrates that women's educational development occurs best in relationship (Belenky, Clinchy, Goldberger, & Tarule, 1986). Mentoring is a relational phenomenon and is, therefore, a natural component of teaching (Vance, 1995). Mentoring emphasizes "caring" as a core value in the teaching-learning enterprise. Mentor relationships with students assist them in tapping into their unique strengths and empower them in their professional and personal lives. The "expectation effect" in mentoring also may prove to be a factor in the outcomes of these relationships (Rosenthal & Jacobson, 1968). The self-fulfilling prophecy, the influence of one person's expectation on another's behavior, can be a powerful component of mentor relationships. If the protégé is treated as someone worthy of assistance and promise, would not this protégé begin to believe in the expectations of the mentor and act on these? Would not the protégé's performance and behavior change as a result of the self-fulfilling prophecy? Will increased self-confidence and self-belief, stemming from the mentor's belief, lead to empowerment and enhanced development of the protégé? The value of these aspects of mentorship is provided by the student perspective as well as that of the leader-mentor. The following story presents a mentor's viewpoint.

The Mentor Connection for Student Leaders

by Robert V. Piemonte

The mentor connection between those of us in leadership positions and students is perhaps the most important contribution that we will make to the profession. Today's students are the profession's legacy. The investment that we make in them is indeed our investment in nursing's future. One problem that I have seen is the lack of mentors. This scarcity exists because so many of us won't take the time to give that extra help to many students who would benefit from this support. There are some basic tenets of mentoring to be followed by those of us in leadership positions. First, it is relatively easy to identify and assist the bright extrovert who hungers for knowledge. The more difficult task is to seek out the bright, but retiring or reluctant students who are less apt to reach out to us. Second, although mentorship in the truest sense is teaching or tutoring, we should not lecture. Rather, a mood should be set that conveys a sharing of information and points of view that the student doesn't have. Third, the student should initiate as many questions and as much dialogue as we, the leaders, do. Finally, mentoring is a long-term commitment. Certain students have "adopted" me. I have mentored them not only as students, but long after they graduated. I truly believe that if we do a good job, we will be continually sought out. The message is simple: Give of yourself to the next generation as a mentor and thereby enrich our proud heritage as a profession and invest in its future strength.

THE GRADUATE STUDENT

Nurses beginning graduate study frequently arrive from a base of clinical expertise to being a novice, both in the classroom and in new role expectations. This process is parallel to that of the undergraduate role development stage. Since they are preparing for new roles in advanced practice, scholarship and research, mentor relationships are essential for graduate students' successful role socialization and development. Mentoring in graduate education is a "unique relationship that is spawned from a mutual perception and experience of need for professional connection, interpersonal growth, scientific inquiry, and theory-based clinical practice (Stewart & Krueger, 1996). Many professors understand that their graduate students will carry the profession into the future, and they want to leave their imprints through their protégés (Budhos, 1996). In academia, this legacy of teacher-student mentoring relations creates something like families—"a kinship because they share a worldview that has been transmitted across the generations" (Gehrke, 1988, p. 193). The graduate student-professor relationship has been described in this way:

> Graduate students are forever changed by the process [of graduate study]. When they emerge, they have joined the fellowship of scholars which remains their main community . . . this is the main job of the graduate professor-mentor—to change a young ward forever and by so doing to ensure his or her own immortality. . . . Scholars believe that what they do matters; their immortality, even though it may be anonymous, is gained through transmission of their heritage through relationships. (Phillips, 1979, p. 345)

Graduate students' mentors are faculty, practicing professionals, and peers (Hanson & Hilde, 1989; Heinrich & Scherr, 1994; Linc & Campbell, 1995; Pardue, 1983). Mentor/preceptor-student relationships in the practice setting are a primary component of graduate education. Committed and experienced mentors in clinical, academic, and research settings facilitate applied learning experiences, student confidence and empowerment, and competence in the specialty area (Hayes & Harrell, 1994; Sealy, 1987; Valadez & Lund, 1993). Weekes (1989) believes that the mentoring process elevates graduate education beyond the acquisition of informational and technical expertise. From the mentor-protégé relationship, graduate students receive support from leaders who can assist with techniques of abstraction and scholarly inquiry in professional issues. A case study of a mentor relationship between a faculty-mentor and a master's student protégé that evolved over a period of several years was described by Stewart and Krueger (1996). They state that their mentor relationship developed because of chemistry and commitment; time investment; their joint productivity in the academic setting; reciprocal career development, research, and scholarship; socialization of the student-protégé into a community of scholars; and their scholarly contribution to concept development in the profession.

Faculty are also instrumental in connecting students with nursing mentors beyond the academic setting, as illustrated in the following vignette.

Mentoring Graduate Nursing Students in Home Health Nursing

by Felicitas A. dela Cruz, Lyvia M. Villegas, and Angeline M. Jacobs

A Graduate Nursing Mentor Program was established in the High Risk Home Health Nursing Clinical Specialty Program at Azusa Pacific University in California to improve the retention and academic success of graduate students who are members of minority ethnic groups. Mentoring partnerships were established between the graduate students and mentors who were minority nursing leaders, such as clinical nurse specialists or leaders in home care nursing. The mentor relationship was formalized for at least 1 year. This pilot program met its objectives, for example, the grade point average of the mentored students was higher than that of nonmentored minority students. The program has been so well received that it will be expanded to all enrolled graduate nursing students. The enduring influence and empowering nature of these relationships are expressed in the evaluation. One mentor stated, "My protégé and I established a close complementary relationship; I have learned from her as well. Our interaction has evolved to one of mutual respect and pride. Graduate study can be very competitive, and mentoring has made me realize the importance of a support system to surmount the challenges. Graduate work can be thus experienced in the spirit of fun and friendship." One of the protégés said, "It was always my dream to attend graduate school. Ten years lapsed since my undergraduate studies, and the academic environment felt foreign and difficult. Thanks to my mentor's encouragement and role modeling, my dream is coming true. My mentor validates my strengths and skills and has taught me to rely on my strengths and lifelong accomplishments. My future plans include pursuing doctoral education in community nursing. I genuinely feel that my mentor's presence in my life has directed me to this end."

An exploratory study was conducted in 1983 by Diane Lancaster to describe the prevalence and characteristics of mentor relationships among newly prepared master's level nurses. She found that the most common mentor function was serving as a positive role model. Encouraging the protégé to believe in himself or herself was also a paramount function. She states that her study and other research demonstrate that advanced practice roles can be developed more easily if mentoring is present from graduate study to the practice arena.

Doctoral students are expected to advance their knowledge and skills in leadership, research, and theory development. The essential contribution of mentoring to scholarship and leadership development during doctoral and postdoctoral study has been discussed by several authors (Ardery, 1990; Davidhizer, 1988; Fitzpatrick & Abraham, 1987; Hinshaw, 1990, 1992; May, Meleis, & Winstead-Fry, 1982; Meleis, 1992; Young, 1985). Since women and nurses are generally newcomers to higher education and doctoral work, the nature of their mentoring relationships in academe is a relatively unexplored territory at the same time that these relationships are of great consequence in their successful development as scholars (Hall & Sandler, 1983; Heinrich, 1995). A study by Olson and Connelly (1995) reported that faculty-doctoral student mentor dyads provided enhancement of the learning experiences beyond course work. In addition, it is increasingly apparent that ensuring scholarly achievement among ethnic minority nurses will require affiliation with and mentoring by the entire nursing community (Bessent, 1989; Valverde, 1980; Waters, 1996).

The promotion of the scholarly development of doctoral students in nursing is described below.

Group as Mentor: Creating Academic Communities of Scholarly Caring

by Kathleen T. Heinrich

Although the concept of "group as mentor" is relatively new, faculty and students can be consciously socialized into collaborative roles through participation in groups that become communities of scholarly caring. In these groups, scholarly caring is demonstrated by creating a safe place for sharing ideas and works in progress, exchanging relevant resources, compassionately reviewing each other's work, and offering honest, constructive feedback. The groups that we created to promote scholarly development through group mentoring include a *qualitative research interest group*, the *hero's journey research project* (Heinrich, Rogers, Haley, & Taylor, 1995), and a *writer's support group*.

The *qualitative research interest group* consisted of faculty and students who were enrolled in or had completed the qualitative research class. This milieu engenders not only an abiding interest in an individual's work, but offers members the opportunity to be mentored for various projects by the best available student or faculty mentors within the group. These collaborative mentoring connections are grounded in an intimate knowledge of each other's work that did not exist between faculty and students prior to the group. The *hero's journey research project* was established to create empowering educational experiences that would strengthen doctoral students' sense of self during their study. Reportedly, women doctoral students often lose their "voice" and sense of self in pursuit of their new identity as scholar-researchers. Experiential workshops and reunions were established to deepen an understanding of participants' graduate transformation into a scholarly identity. This new identity evolved out of the dialectic between self-reliance and connectedness with the group. Participants developed their "scholarly voice" within the context of a group that over time became a community of "scholarly caring" (Meleis, Hall, & Stevens, 1994). The *writer's support group*, consisting of faculty and students, involved mutual feedback on writing samples, peer editing, sharing of relevant resources, as well as mutual feedback in a group mentoring framework.

Some may argue that the very notion of "group as mentor" dilutes the meaning of the mentor concept. Sadly, the mystique of exclusive, one-to-one mentoring relationships has divided nurses into the "haves" and the "have nots" for too long. Creating communities of scholarly caring among faculty and students makes it possible for all involved to give and receive mentoring. Collaborative mentoring in faculty-student groups has the potential for reinstating the "matrilineal lines of initiation—older women teaching younger women—that have long been fragmented and broken" (Estes, 1992, p. 264). The hope is that feminist nurse educators, researchers, and students—women and men—will together create ways to extend mentoring to each other through the continued development of "group as mentor."

In summary, students engaged in graduate study must confront a paradigm shift in their professional commitment and values, devise different methodologies for conceptualizing and applying knowledge, give up the role of "expert" to become again a "novice," and find a new "voice" and new ways of knowing. Mentor connections throughout this paradigm shift can provide a solid foundation of encouragement and support for a successful transition to leadership roles and excellence in scholarship and advanced practice.

MENTOR PROGRAMS FOR STUDENTS

The establishment of formal mentor programs in schools of nursing is becoming prevalent as the benefits are documented. Professional career socialization, personal growth, educational and career achievement, and leadership development are cited benefits of these programs. Educational institutions can provide mentoring assistance through a variety of alternatives, including formal programs (Hall & Sandler, 1983). In a longitudinal study of retention and its relationship to the emotional, social, and academic adjustment of college students, it was pointed out that faculty mentoring programs and small special interest seminars taught by faculty contribute to overall student retention (Gerdes & Mallinckrodt, 1994). For example, the Faculty Mentoring Program for minority undergraduate students in a large California university was found to contribute to high academic performance and enhanced retention and graduation rates (Gonzalez, 1994).

Dee Baldwin and Judith Wold established the Nursing Mentor Program, originally for students from disadvantaged backgrounds, at Georgia State University in 1991. The primary goal of the program is student retention; other goals include the promotion of leadership, scholarship, and professional skill development. For the program, mentoring is defined as the sustained interaction between faculty-peer mentors and student protégés in an academic setting. The mentor relationship focuses on the lived experience of both faculty and students as they engage in the mentoring process, that is, how the faculty and students listen and respond to each other. The five programmatic components are (a) recruitment, (b) quarterly program meetings, (c) a summer enrichment course, (d) mentor-protégé sessions, and (e) faculty and student development. Through evaluation studies, the program has been found to foster confidence, self-esteem, and motivation among the students. Many students in the program are serving in leadership positions in the school and college (Baldwin & Wold, 1993b; Wold, 1993). Student retention has improved, and the program received the Best Practices in Retention Award from the University System of Georgia in 1996. Baldwin and Wold state:

> The greatest strength of the Nursing Mentor Program is its promotion of the belief in the capabilities of the students. Simply, the program holds forth the expectation that students are capable of learning complex materials at a high skill level. Students are not only expected to pass the course work, but to excel. As a result of this philosophy in our mentoring, many students in the program have developed leadership skills and hold leadership positions both in the school and [the] community. As one protégé stated, "We are expected to be leaders!"

The San Jose State University School of Nursing in California has a substantial percentage of minority students and has in place a Nurse Mentor Program that matches minority nursing students with minority nurse mentors and peers. Katherine Abriam-Yago, coordinator of the program, describes its approach:

> I have found that the two primary areas of need with minority students are emotional support and interpersonal communication skills. Originally funded by a state grant, 43 students were matched with nurse mentors. Many students reported increased feelings of security, reduction of anxiety levels, and improvement of grades that they attributed to the positive influence and support provided by the mentors. The relationship helped them to focus on the goal of becoming a nurse, raised their self-esteem, and enhanced their nursing skills. Students also reported increased motivation to do their best when matched with a nurse mentor who shared the same background. They gained insight into the realities of nursing practice and career choices, and saw their mentors as excellent role models. We have found that for the mentor relationship to be successful, a commitment must be established

between the mentors and students. Both must be open to change and willing to commit time and energy required in the relationship. Although sometimes challenging, we have found that mentors make a significant difference in the retention, ability, and satisfaction of minority nursing students. It is also a very rewarding partnership.

The Ethnic Minority R.N. Mentor Project at Ohlone College in Fremont, California, engages ethnic registered nurses from the community as mentors with traditionally at-risk students early in their nursing education. Data analysis reveals similar findings at other programs. Bernadette VanDeusen reports that the attrition rate of students in the program is only 8%, lower that the school's average. Student-mentors' social support networks have expanded, and their perception of social support has increased. Upon graduation, they are eager to mentor students, wanting to give back what they have received. Mentors report enjoying watching their protégés succeed. On occasion, they support them through failure. They feel they have made a difference and see it as an opportunity to give back to the profession and to their own ethnic group. Some mentors express a new sense of pride in their professional work. VanDeusen reports the following factors that she believes ensure success in a formal program:

- being well matched, having similar backgrounds;
- geographic proximity;
- clear expectations at the beginning of the relationship;
- voluntary participation;
- a feeling of being treated with consideration and respect in the relationship;
- a feeling of the relationship being valued by both parties;
- an available institutional liaison whom they feel comfortable talking with;
- attending on-campus get-togethers sponsored by the institution; and
- being acknowledged by the institution for one's efforts.

My Mentor

by Dianna P. Ross

I enrolled in a nursing program when I was 17, and although I am a very independent person, there were times when I needed help. I remember the first time I asked for help from a faculty member who was nice but was too busy to help me. I didn't take it personally, but I prided myself on never having to ask for help. After this experience, I decided I should try even harder on my own. Then I met Ms. Lucia Rusty, who told me about the Mentor Program at the university. After she explained to me what a mentor was and what he or she does, I gave this opportunity serious thought and decided that a mentor could help me with decision making. Ms. Rusty paired me with Ms. Ventryce Thomas at Stony Brook Hospital in New York. I could see that as an administrator she was an extremely busy person, so I didn't expect too much of her time. However, I quickly felt that she was someone I could trust and feel comfortable with. After several meetings and a tour of her hospital, I knew that finally I had found someone whom I could talk with about nursing and anything that was bothering me. I told Ms. Rusty that Ms. Thomas was the perfect mentor. She was always there for me to talk to and would take my phone calls no matter how busy she was. At the end of the year, I learned that students can nominate their mentors for "The Mentor of the Year Award" and write essays about them. My winning essay allowed Ms. Thomas to receive the award at a reception. When she walked onto the stage to accept the award, it was one of the best days of my life. It made me happy to see the smile on her face and hear the joy in her voice. I was just pleased that I could do a little something for my mentor, who has done so much for me.

My Role as Mentor

by Ventryce Thomas

My entire professional career has been involved with mentoring. In the late 1970s, I sponsored students from five high schools in Queens, New York. As the director of a hospital staff education program, I interviewed and selected the students and mentored them through various departments in the hospital each semester. One of my high school protégés is now a vice president for nursing and a doctoral candidate. He told me that his first career choice was to be a physician, but he had me in his mind as a model and changed his career path to nursing. I was invited to participate in the formal mentor program at Stony Brook University and have been involved in that program for more than 6 years in spite of a hectic work schedule. With Dianna and two other students, I have tried very hard to assist them, seeking out people with expertise to help where I couldn't. My protégés are still connected with me. I was really shocked but very pleased when I was given the mentor award. It has been the highest honor bestowed upon me, and I am truly grateful. Young people are honest. They are not hypocritical. They feel deeply, and for Dianna to feel this way really touched me. I see my protégés as family, like nieces and nephews. I hold them to high expectations with deep affection. It is my hope that when they get older, they will become mentors to others. I enjoy the mentor role and feel that as nurses, we need to mentor our students. We can all learn from each other.

The Mentor Program

by Lucia M. Rusty

The Mentor Program at Stony Brook University in New York was established in 1984 to encourage and motivate undergraduate students to excel in their studies and persist to graduation. The seeds for this program were planted by three high-achieving students who requested that they have their own special person, a professional with whom to develop a personal-support relationship while matriculating in college. The program currently has about 360 mentors and 340 student protégés, the majority being female and from minority backgrounds. Mentors share their knowledge, wisdom, life experiences and information about the university. It is hoped that these relationships will ensure greater success for the protégés as they meet the challenges of college and transition into their life's career. The size and longevity of Mentor Program can be attributed to the university's administrative and fiscal support and the active voluntary involvement of faculty, staff, and professional volunteer mentors, as well as the participation of students who treasure the mentoring experience.

There are variations of these student mentor programs, particularly in the mentor population. For example, Nancy DeBasio describes a mentor-protégé program for senior nursing students that was established between a medical center and a college of nursing. Evaluation of the program revealed several areas of concern among the nurse-mentors and student-protégés including lack of sufficient time to work together, lack of interpersonal skills on the part of either mentor or protégé, unrealistic expectations, and an overdependence on the mentor. Appropriate modifications have been made. Six years later, the program has been extended to include nurse-mentors from additional acute care settings as well as community agencies and long-term care facilities. The mentor dyads are now initiated in the spring of the students' sophomore year, which allows the development of an extended relationship. Program goals and expectations are provided in a more extensive orientation, and subsequent group sessions are held. Dr. DeBasio believes that the strength of the profession and the optimism necessary to move it forward lie in the collaborative efforts of practice and education in the form of mentor-protégé programs and partnerships. The alumni of schools also are getting involved as mentors to the students of their alma maters. This approach is described in the following story.

Caring for Each Other: The Student and Alumni Mentor Connection

by Penny Bamford, Russell Hullstrung, and Mary Plitsas

The Mentor Connection Program at the College of New Rochelle School of Nursing in New York involves students and graduates of their alma mater. This program was begun as a pilot program in the late 1980s with 17 dyads of alumni and students at all levels. The lessons learned from the pilot included the need for improved matching criteria, increased structure, consideration of time constraints, and additional institutional support. The current program has over 70 mentor-protégé dyads. Interviews were conducted with a selected sample to elucidate the experience of being a protégé or mentor. The words of the participants evolved as themes that, when woven together, form a description and meaning of the mentor connection. These were themes of teaching-learning, guidance-support, and reflection-insight. These are the reciprocal, dynamic, and organizing structures of the mentor connection.

The mentor connection of caring has eased difficult situations—situations that result in behaviors reflective of issues of values, ethics, and race, conflict management, and self-awareness. These issues are related to oppressed-group behavior; some are due to inadequate communication and conflict resolution skills, and a basic need to learn how to deal with one's feelings in relation to life situations and appropriate management of those feelings. Clinical nursing interventions focus on helping clients cope, providing support, and caring deeply about them. Our obligation also extends beyond our clients to include ourselves, our students, and our colleagues in the development of nurturing relationships that result in the growth of each individual. We struggle with these issues, knowing that resolution of them is beyond the traditional modes of teaching, learning, and socialization. We wish that we and our students will experience an increased connectedness to our school and profession, and that we might individually and collectively develop self-determination, self-sufficiency, and inner-directedness. The Mentor Connection Program was initiated in response to this wish and has been a motivating framework for reciprocal growth for all of us. The next steps include the development of evaluation criteria, additional training for both mentors and protégés, and program expansion to include student-peer mentoring and faculty-faculty mentoring.

In summary, as students are introduced and socialized to the profession, their experiences can be shaped and strengthened by experienced nurse-mentors. Faculty, established professionals, alumni, and peers who are willing to give the gifts of time and emotional commitment to these developing professionals share their legacy for the future of the profession.

THE FACULTY

Many novice nursing faculty appear on the doorstep of academe with clinical expertise and credentials but without knowledge of the academic culture. Teaching and scholarship skills frequently need honing, as well as guidance with the balancing of multiple role demands (Megel, 1985). Although mentoring is not a panacea for every academic challenge, newcomers to academe, often outside the "inner circle," such as women and minorities, can benefit greatly from the support of established academics or professionals in their fields of study.

A survey of the frequency, quality, and influence of mentoring among faculty (N = 1,234) in a northern California university is reported by Carol Huston. She relates that 61% of respondents claimed a significant faculty-faculty mentoring relationship at the university, with an average length of 3 to 5 years. Ms. Huston found that male faculty generally mentored male faculty, and female faculty generally mentored female faculty. As a result of male dominance in high-level university ranks and the gender-specific nature of mentoring, male faculty have a greater opportunity for participation in a mentoring relationship, and mentoring of female faculty is limited because of the decreased availability of senior female faculty mentors. She says:

> In any case, mentoring was viewed by an overwhelming majority of respondents, male and female, as a powerful tool for the retention, tenure and promotion of junior faculty, particularly women. Mentor relationships among faculty support the faculty-protégé in scholarly endeavors, but more important, assist the protégé to understand and break through the political and social barriers within the department, school or faculty group. Study findings suggest that mentorship in academe provides benefits similar to those reported in corporate settings: advancement, achievement, and socialization.

Women in the academy face special challenges. Despite much progress, many patterns have not changed in relation to women faculty's rank, tenure, and salary. Sandler (1993) discusses the structural, psychological, and sociological explanations for women's lack of progress. Because of these factors, she believes that networking and mentoring relationships are essential for both survival and success of women academics. Collegiate and university schools of nursing, with a predominance of women faculty, are increasingly implementing mentoring through formal programs to assist faculty in the primary role components of teaching, service, and research.

A Model for Mentoring Junior Nursing Faculty

by Regina M. Sallee Williams

The Department of Nursing Education at Eastern Michigan University has formalized a mentoring model in which senior faculty mentor junior faculty to facilitate achievement of reappointment, tenure, promotion, and scholarly work. In this program, faculty mentors are committed to mentoring a novice faculty member, to share their expertise in areas of mutual interest, and to meet on a regular basis to assist him or her in becoming familiar with the culture of the university, college, and department. The purposes of this mentorship are to: (a) provide new faculty members with a support structure that facilitates learning about the academic culture; (b) help the faculty member attain the rewards of reappointment, tenure, and promotion; and (c) assist faculty without the doctoral degree to complete the degree and those with the doctoral degree to pursue their scholarship. Senior nursing faculty members are assigned to newly hired faculty, and senior faculty from other disciplines also serve as mentors to nursing faculty who are interested in a particular research methodology or population. Junior faculty are encouraged to develop their scholarly work and to focus on building a cohesive research program. In spite of the requisite time commitment, we believe that the program is an important investment. The colleagueship that develops during these mentoring relationships has far-reaching ramifications for academic success and satisfaction, scholarly productivity, and professional commitment.

A similar program at Nassau Community College in New York pairs new and tenured faculty in the Department of Nursing. Mentors assist new faculty members in incorporating the philosophy and objectives of the nursing program into the classroom and clinical learning experiences. Roseanna Mills, Jane Brody and Thora Heeseler report that for new faculty, the mentoring process includes several facets: assistance with classroom lectures and materials; support with clinical supervision; and information sharing about the day-to-day functioning of the department and college. They note that "an equally important but less quantifiable aspect of the mentoring process is the assurance for new faculty that they are not overlooked or not valued—that there is someone who is committed to serving as their mentor and resource person to whom they can turn for advice and guidance."

Male nursing faculty and their mentor relationships were investigated by Clark (1994). Sixty-seven percent of the study population (N = 114) reported that they had been mentored, mainly by female nurses. There was not a significant difference in scholarly productivity between mentored and nonmentored male faculty. Clark reports that in this study, in contrast to other studies, the male protégés initiated the mentor relationships. She states that while studies of male mentoring demonstrate that the most satisfying relationships were same-gender relationships, rewarding cross-gender mentor relationships also can occur as with these male protégés and their female mentors. Further, she believes that if female nurse educators were more active in initiating mentoring relationships, male protégés would benefit greatly from their involvement. She deems that "although it is probably easier for women to approach women in initiating mentor relationships than it is for women to approach men, we must move beyond this behavior. We should examine our perceptions of men as colleagues and embrace the mentor role more actively with them."

THE ACADEMIC ADMINISTRATOR

Studies show that the academic dean must wear many hats, balance various priorities, and be sensitive to and support faculty, staff, and student needs (Kavoosi, Elman, & Mauch, 1995; Vance, 1995). Nursing deans can motivate faculty to commitment and leadership, thus shaping the future of their schools and ultimately the profession (Larson, 1994). Their mentorship of various constituencies should be a critical component of their leadership. Academic administrators also need mentors. In a study of deans, Lamborn (1991) reported that only 50% had any formal preparation for this role. To achieve and maintain success and satisfaction in this complex role, sustained mentor relationships and formal preparation are crucial. Collaborative mentoring in which greater numbers of academic leaders, faculty and students mentor each other will transform the academy and the discipline of nursing. This is truly transformational leadership in which "leaders and followers raise one another to higher levels of motivation and morality" (Burns, 1978, p. 20).

Reflections of Mentors: Nurse Leaders in Academe

by Mary Boose Walker

I began my mentoring journey as a new faculty member and doctoral student at the University of Pennsylvania 20 years ago. Our dean, Dr. Claire Fagin, a nurse-influential and scholar, possessed a leadership style characterized by "star making" and mentoring for success. Her assumption was that women, including nurses in academe, would succeed by moving up the hierarchy, just as they could in the corporate world. This was a time of affirmative action, of minorities and women demanding admission to "the club," claiming their rightful places in top academic positions, and climbing the ladder to previously all-male bastions of power and privilege. Now as an academic administrator, I reflect upon three lessons my journey taught me:

1. Legislated equal opportunity—while a critical starting point—is not enough. Mentors are necessary for leadership success.
2. The traditional mentor-protégé dyadic model is insufficient for the challenges we face.
3. A new paradigm for caring and scholarship must emerge.

This new paradigm redefines success as enabling others to succeed in a turbulent, diverse world of global villages; engages faculty and students as mutual teachers and learners outside the walls of academe; and the consumer acts as the sage mentor, helping health care professionals understand that looking through the telescope of someone else's experiences can alter perceptions (Walker & Frank, 1995).

One recurring theme in my studies about women leaders (Walker, 1981, 1984) is the value of their mentor connections and networks for sharing traditions, beliefs, values, and wisdom. Does mentoring have to be the ubiquitous, often isolating dyadic model that has existed since the time of Homer? I believe that we can change the rules and create a new vision of mentorship based on collaboration and community. I want a new paradigm for empowering nursing leaders and scholars for caring in changing times, one that transcends politics as usual. A paradigm must emerge that reframes success as enabling others to succeed. My vision of the future is a collaborative, inclusive one that welcomes diversity; it is a global mosaic of collective wisdom, gleaned from sages of all ages—a collective wisdom that will allow future leaders to soar confidently on wings of ambiguity and change. Our new, evolving mentor relationships will be central to this vision of collaboration and community.

7

Mentoring in the Practice Setting

What has happened to the art of mentorship? Why don't senior nurses reach out to help young staff who are so obviously in need of strong support? And, conversely, why don't young nurses seek that counsel instead of isolating themselves in a web of anxiety? When the young don't seek and the mature don't offer, both are deprived (Thelma Schorr, 1979).

Most nurses practice the science and art of nursing and healing in clinical organizations. The journey from being a novice practitioner to becoming an expert is the developmental imperative. Establishing organizational climates in which this journey creates empowerment and excellence in professional practice is the challenge of leaders. Mentor connections assist in the development of knowledge and skills at each professional stage, and ultimately of excellence in nursing practice. Caring and healing relationships among practitioners, as evidenced in their mentor relationships, enable them to establish caring and healing relationships with their patients as well.

THE NOVICE

Nurses in the clinical setting increasingly recognize the need to mentor neophyte nurses as they begin their clinical practice. Although nursing historically has not utilized formal internships and residencies, new practitioners are introduced to the profession through various forms of preceptorships, staff orientation, and development programs. Preceptors, staff educators, and experienced clinicians have served as mentors to apprentice-nurses. Sociologists have described the essential role of the "master-apprentice" relationship in the professions and the sciences through which initiation, identification, and transmission of the central tenets of the discipline occur. The phenomenon of sponsorship in the established professions has been the way in which junior persons move forward in their work and profession through the involvement of a more established person (Becker & Strauss, 1956). Learning the complex practice of nursing necessitates this guided sponsorship by experienced and interested mentors. The shared responsibility of cultivating mentor relationships to bridge the gap between nursing education and practice will result in a more satisfied and better prepared nurse population and thereby a more satisfied consumer-patient (Beaulieu, 1988).

In a health care climate characterized by a volatile supply and demand of professional nurses, particularly in the hospital setting, the mentorship model is being adopted to bring new nurses into the system and to retain and support them in delivering high-quality care. At New York University Medical Center, for example, a Nurse Residency Program was initiated in the spring of 1996 to provide an intensive, mentored, clinical experience for new graduates of baccalaureate programs. Modeled after the 2-year Clinical Entry Nurse Residency Program at Beth Israel Hospital in Boston, this 1-year program assists new graduates to become competent practitioners with knowledge, skills, and flexibility to practice in any clinical setting across the continuum of care. New York University's Nurse Residency Program is a proactive response to the recognition that changes in the health care environment also have changed the expectations and the role of the registered nurse. The novice nurses are assigned mentors to socialize and support them in their professional role identity, facilitate their entry into the practice setting, and introduce them to nursing practice in a highly acute, tertiary care setting. Among other features, clinically enriched conference days are planned with the nurse resident, the mentor, and the coordinator of the program that provide customized experiences focusing on the broader scope of patient care required in today's environment.

Dr. Susan Bowar-Ferres, senior administrator and director of nursing, explains that the nurse residents in this program are paid slightly

less than the regular entry staff nurse and receive full employee benefits. At the completion of the residency program, the nurse can apply
for a senior staff nurse position, although a position is not guaranteed.
Dr. Bowar-Ferres emphasizes that the nurse-mentors get more deeply
involved in a wider array of professional issues with their protégés
than a preceptor would, including guidance, coaching, counseling,
nurturing, and role modeling beyond the unit role. The Nurse Residency
Program, incorporating mentorship, has been so successful as a pilot
that the model is being implemented with all new B.S.N. graduates.
The anecdotal evidence of a more global perspective of nursing's role
in the continuum of care, heightened critical thinking skills, and
greater initiative has supported the institutional decision to implement
this program more extensively. Prospective comparisons of selected
variables demonstrated by nurse residents and traditional new staff
nurses will be conducted as the program progresses.

A small, quasi-experimental study of the effects of providing mentors for B.S.N. graduate nurses revealed that significant differences
existed in several areas of job satisfaction and in perceived leadership
behaviors in the experimental and control groups. Job retention also
was improved (Hamilton, Murray, Lindholm, & Myers, 1989). Another
study of new graduates using a mentoring model was conducted by
the Medical Nursing Service at the Johns Hopkins University Hospital.
Two dimensions of mentor relationships—career and psychosocial—
as described by Yoder (1990) were investigated. Mary Alice Johnson,
Maria Cvach, and Valerie Parks discuss their findings:

> We found that units with new graduate nurses who partici-
> pate in formal mentor programs have higher retention rates
> than those who do not. New graduates who participate in a
> formal mentor program have a greater increase in job satisfac-
> tion that those who do not. Since informal mentoring occurs
> in addition to the formal mentor program, the Mentor Task
> Force is attempting to create an environment that incorporates
> mentoring in various aspects of nursing practice, including
> orientation and preceptor workshops, clinical nurse advance-
> ment programs, nursing care delivery model planning, and
> clinical ladder advancement. We believe that mentoring rela-
> tionships will flourish in this environment. The hospital is
> undergoing re-engineering and transitioning into a new care
> delivery model, and mentoring will be incorporated into the
> leading of a high performance team.

With the intensive incorporation of managed care in the health care industry, every discipline must examine its practice in a cost-quality perspective. Appropriate socialization, professional commitment, and satisfaction of the practitioner will be necessary to deliver efficient, high quality, cost-effective care. Mary Cooper says:

> Retention and work satisfaction can be achieved by employing a system-wide mentorship that promotes a culture of professional development, open communication, conflict resolution, and participative management. These ingredients produce high-quality patient care—the cornerstone of the health care industry—by highly developed nurses who are committed and satisfied with their work. We have developed a management system, utilizing mentoring as a major building block, which has evolved into a shared governance model and staff empowerment. The culture of a nursing unit begins with shared values. If the values are individualization or competitiveness, then mentoring one another does not succeed. If the manager has a vision of building a team where each person's development is central and where people can take risks without fear of reprisal and can resolve conflict directly, then a culture of mentoring can occur.

THE ADVANCED PRACTICE NURSE

There is a growing public demand for advanced practice nurses who engage in high-level assessment and decision making, clinical interventions, and research utilization with patients presenting complex needs. The advanced practice role includes that of the clinician, teacher, leader, manager, consultant, change agent, research or theory implementer, and evaluator (Hamilton et al., 1990; Hupcey, 1990). The evolutionary role of these practitioners requires graduate preparation and the exquisite guidance, direction, and nurturing of experienced mentors (Hanson & Hilde, 1989; Hockenberry-Eaton & Kline, 1995). Eileen Hayes makes the case for the crucial role of mentoring in promoting self-efficacy of advanced practice nurses:

> Self-efficacy is a personal conviction and self-confidence in one's ability to accomplish a goal or task. Mentor relationships promote self-efficacy, for it is the mentor who recognizes the potential of the novice, instills confidence and

provides opportunities for new experiences. Mentoring involves much more of an extended commitment and investment from agencies than the traditional precepting model. This is a valuable investment, as it is the mentoring experience that can ultimately assist in the development of more efficacious providers who can make significant contributions, particularly in primary care. Learning to appreciate the patient's lived experience does not happen easily or quickly. The mentor relationship over time could be the most effective way to accomplish this skill. Assuring an adequate supply of competent advanced practice nurses requires promoting awareness of their need for mentoring, developing mentor programs based on a nursing model, finding ways to reward mentoring, nurturing future mentors who will mentor others, assisting students and practitioners in mentor-seeking, and demonstrating the relationship between mentoring and self-efficacy through research.

Benner (1984) believes that the "relational, interpretive, and coaching functions of nurses are increasingly recognized as central to patient recovery and health promotion" (p. 145). Hearing the patient's voice may be the most important contribution of the practitioner. This is accomplished by listening to the perceived concerns of the patient, by the use of a shared language and a stance of copartnership, and by conversation that establishes a connectedness to "patient talk" (Johnson, 1993). These communication competencies are learned through collegial mentor relationships that serve as models for patient-nurse relationships.

The mentoring role with patients is described by Dr. Karen Forbes, a family nurse practitioner:

I believe that all teaching and learning occur in relationship, which is especially true in graduate education and advanced clinical nursing practice. As a nurse practitioner, I must make sense out of, and therapeutically intervene in, complex and confusing clinical situations. My mentoring role in the nurse practitioner-patient relationship is central to my practice. I work with individuals and their families who suffer with the chronic disease of diabetes that requires considerable patient/family involvement, patient control and shared treatment responsibility with me. They are unwilling sufferers and have this disease in a culture that promotes passive treatment by medication. In my opinion, this is the ultimate in the mentor-protégé relationship, for it usually takes months and years to develop, often only after complications occur. Initially the patient-protégé usually does not want and resents the need for this relationship. As the nurse practitioner, diabetes educator, and mentor, my role is to listen carefully; stimulate learning, coping and self-development skills; teach self-care skills needed to live with diabetes; and assist the patient in adopting lifestyle changes that are health promoting, often while grieving and denying the diagnosis. Our relationship hopefully engages the patient and family in acquiring the hope and self-confidence that they can live with the disease. Mutually, when this relationship works, we both gain in increased self-esteem as we realize that our mutual and shared work has improved a person's and family's health. We mutually encourage and support each other. I facilitate their continued control of their diabetes, and they allow me to know that I can make a positive difference in my patients' lives. It is the ultimate reward to have patients return with improved health care and glycemic indexes, a positive outlook, a feeling of control in their lives, and satisfaction with their perceived improved health. Sometimes, however, no matter how hard I try with some patients, I cannot seem to make a difference. I do not give up, but I also must realize that the mentor relationship depends on the mutuality of both persons. To me, mentor-practitioner and protégé-patient relationships consist of mutual respect, collaboration, and mutual growth through commitment and hard work.

Mentor relationships in nursing practice cannot always be quantified and understood from a scientific perspective. The essence of true mentor-nurse and protégé-patient relationships lies within their existential foundation. They are a form of the "I-Thou" relationship that occurs simply because these two persons are who they are, and their relationship serves to develop the total presence of both individuals (Vaillot, 1966). These relationships highlight the significance of the less quantifiable aspects of nursing care, such as mobilizing hope, active listening to patient's concerns, energizing patient involvement, eliciting the support of significant others, and negotiating mutual goals in

a holistic context (Brykczynski, 1993). These outcomes are best elucidated through qualitative investigation.

THE CLINICAL LEADER

The contemporary complexities of a changing health care system,
restructured organizations, and global relationships require leaders
who value connectedness, collaboration, flexibility, and empowerment
of others. These qualities, frequently valued and possessed by women
leaders, will be very advantageous to nursing professionals and will
lead naturally to mentoring among each other. A major responsibility
of leaders is to develop people. Leaders influence others to work
toward common goals and to develop to their fullest potential. This
means that the leader is a teacher and a mentor. Learning relationships
(Haynor, 1994) and career development relationships (Yoder, 1990,
1992, 1995) that include mentoring are not only essential for the success and satisfaction of leaders and followers in the organization but
for the development and well-being of the entire organization.

In today's clinical world, nursing managers and executives must
not only embrace change but create it. In the midst of sometimes
chaotic and confusing change, environments must be created where
nurses can care for patients and families and for each other (Wright,
1995). Nurse executives have a special obligation and opportunity to
engage in this work. Barbara Farley describes the creation of environments for developing others as "passing the baton." She says,

> Throughout my nursing career, I have been incredibly fortu-
> nate. The reason is that from the first day in my first position
> to the present, I have been coached and mentored by wonder-
> ful people. Most were nurses, but not all. The relationship
> with some began by accident and some by design. Those rela-
> tionships are still very precious to me. I have no doubt that I
> would not be in my present position but for the gift of men-
> toring. Now I am the nurse executive in a large academic
> teaching hospital which offers many opportunities to mentor
> people. It is also important to bring the concept to all of the
> nursing professionals on our staff, beginning with the nurse
> managers. We have succeeded in changing our environment
> to a large degree through mentorship. As a leader I open the
> door, give permission, and show the way. But it is the nurses

who make it happen through their caring for each other in the midst of often difficult and challenging work. When nurses mentor nurses, they are not only the winners but their patients as well. Importantly, our nurses have shown that they will continue to pass the mentoring baton among each other.

Nurse managers are often the front-line change agents and are, therefore, in a position to make a substantial difference in the delivery of care. The centrality of mentorship in making change is illustrated in the following story.

The Head Nurse, Mentorship, Leadership, and Change

by Jane O'Malley

As a head nurse responsible for major change in a respiratory care unit, I endeavored to involve the staff in every step of the change process. This approach entailed group and individual mentoring. In my view, leadership is influence; and mentorship is professional support and guidance. I recognize the importance of both in the change process. Mentoring on behalf of change in my unit included teaching, coaching, role modeling, support, advice, and guidance. These are essential tools of staff development and are required of the new breed of leader. I learned these skills from those who so generously mentored and continue to mentor me. I hope I have passed them on to others. In this change situation, the protégé was the group of unit nurses, rather than an individual. Communication is a vital part of the mentoring process, and we paid a lot of attention to how we as a group and as individuals communicated with each other. Continuous dialogue and ownership also are essential elements in the change process. As time passed, it became clear that the nurses were changing in response to their new roles and the support they felt. My role changed reciprocally, becoming one of adviser-mentor rather than director. I guided rather than directed, listening to problems and encouraging group problem solving. Consensus was the method by which we adopted new initiatives. The role-modeling component of mentorship became increasingly important as the nurses struggled with their newfound autonomy. In many instances, the mentoring was individualized. Less experienced nurses needed additional support and guidance. They needed coaching to approach potential conflict situations and benefited from positive reinforcement when completing challenging projects.

My successful experience provides lessons that may be useful to those who mentor in the midst of massive change. First, mentoring provides support and a presence that can reduce feelings of isolation in the face of uncertainty and risk taking. The mentor can provide a sounding board and safety net while pushing hitherto unattainable boundaries. Second, the mentor can assist in speeding up the change process. The mentor can provide warnings of the pitfalls so that predictable mistakes can be avoided. The certainty that comes with experience can be applied to support those who are learning the ropes and to make the process easier. Finally, the mentor assists in the goal-setting and evaluation process of change. The mentor may provide the peg in the ground, the yardstick by which progress is measured. The peg is moved forward to challenge and to allow the protégé to look back and feel encouraged about future possibilities. As someone who has had the good fortune to be mentored, I can attest to the power of the mentoring process in driving change. Having experienced and appreciated the benefits, I was able to act confidently as a mentor to others. I am grateful for both opportunities of receiving and giving mentoring.

Dr. Harriet Forman, who has been a nurse executive for many years, believes that mentoring is a special form of companionship between human beings—a communion that transcends bias and diminishes competition. "I've learned that mentoring seems to be second nature to those who mentor. It's not always something they think about or consciously set out to do. More likely, it comes as a natural extension of their nature, their humanity, their generosity, and their willingness to help. On reflection, administrative mentorship at its core involves taking a deep personal interest in creating an environment for the success of another human being."

To summarize, Diana Weaver offers her perspectives on leadership and mentorship in the clinical setting;

From the protégé's viewpoint, the key themes of the mentor transaction with the nursing leader are shared vision and values; a commitment to lifelong learning; affirmation of the protégé's ability to succeed with increasingly difficult challenges; empowerment; nonjudgmental interactions; shared analysis of complex situations; and guiding principles. It is clear that those who are mentored will mentor others. Those who are mentored internalize that experience as an important element in their own leadership style. Finally, I believe that there are consistent attributes of a mentor relationship that transcend time, place and role.

8

Mentoring for Scholarship and Research Development

It is from my mentors and proteges that I have come to believe that mentorship is the single most sacred and significant variable in the development of scholars and in the progress that we want in our discipline (Afaf Ibrahim Meleis).

For the nursing discipline to reach its full potential, its scientific and research base must be strengthened and expanded. The need for the presence of mentorship to support nursing research productivity has been emphasized by many people in the discipline. The common denominator in scientific advances, according to Dr. Jacqueline Fawcett and Dr. Ruth McCorkle, is a mentor who encourages the scientist to think about questions in the discovery process.

Mentors and Advances in Nursing Science

by Jacqueline Fawcett and Ruth McCorkle

It is our view that mentors are needed throughout a scientist's professional life, that mentors play different roles at different times in a scientist's life, and that mentors are a catalyst for scientific productivity. Mentoring behaviors do not often come naturally within the context of the personal and professional demands of one's life. We, therefore, propose four roles that mentor-scientists can play in advancing nursing science and in mentoring other nurses. These are *teacher, assessor, colleague*, and *coauthor*.

The *mentor-teacher* is important to the student, the neophyte researcher, and the established scientist who wants to expand research into new areas. Typically, the mentor-teacher promotes the protégé's work by being a sponsor, benefactor, protector, supporter, adviser, advocate, and role model. The mentor-teacher brings the protégé into the community of established scientists, recommending the protégé for a choice postdoctoral fellowship and faculty position, and sponsoring the protégé for membership in honorary societies and national committees. The protégé may be taking courses with or working on the mentor-teacher's research team or laboratory. The protégé turns to the mentor-teacher for advice about positions, current and projected work, and the political climate of the scientific community.

The *mentor-assessor* reviews and discusses the scientist's ongoing work, critiques drafts and grant proposals and publications, and offers advice and support. The mentor-assessor acts as a friendly critic who is sought by the scientist because of his or her expertise. Their objective appraisal of the scientist's work is especially valued.

The *mentor-colleague* acts as a collaborator and consultant to new and established nurse scientists. Together they plan and implement problem-solving strategies in a milieu of sharing that overcomes defensive postures and promotes openness to each other's suggestions (Kelly, 1979). Colleagues are enormously important because typically they are involved in the same or closely related programs and can understand the various theoretical, clinical, and methodological aspects of the work. The most highly prized mentor-colleagues are those who are constructively critical of the work as it progresses, for although nurse scientists need support and encouragement, they benefit most from continual, constructive critical reviews of their thoughts and the products of those thoughts.

The *mentor-coauthor* shares the burden and the joy of writing and publishing. Mentor-coauthors may be one or more new scientists who work with the mentor to jointly report research findings, theoretical frames of reference, or methodological approaches. Mentor-coauthors may also be two or more established scientists or a combination of new and established scientists.

The current generation of nurse scientists has directed considerable energy toward initiating and sustaining research programs. The survival and success of these nurse scientists has involved long work hours, painstaking professional advocacy, networking with colleagues from various disciplines, and establishing careful definitions of the domain and mission of nursing science. Often, little time has been available to consider how to best cultivate and nurture the next generation of nurse scientists. The increased interest in mentoring relationships as a vehicle for advancing the research agenda of the discipline as well as the research careers of nurses is a direct result of a cadre of established nurse scientists now in place and the rapid growth of doctoral programs in nursing. Although the activities associated with the four roles initially imply effort by the mentor and benefit for the protégé, both can grow and develop substantially from the mentor relationship. The discipline of nursing and its research and science base will also grow and develop by active mentorship.

The need for mentoring for research development to strengthen the profession also is emphasized by Dr. Dorothy Brooten. She posits that mentoring for research development, while sharing common characteristics with mentoring in education and practice, is unique for two reasons. First, there are fewer research mentors available. Second, the time required to produce an independent investigator is far longer than that required to produce an independent practitioner or educator. The process of mentoring, however, is much the same in that it always includes teaching, guiding, counseling, role modeling, nurturing, and building independence. Dr. Brooten points out that there are only about 9,000 doctorally prepared nurses in the United States, with about 20%–25% of them actually conducting research; hence there is an insufficient number of nurse researchers to meet the current demand in academic and clinical settings for mentoring other researchers. She believes that this situation needs greater discussion and action within the nursing discipline if mentorship in research is to be enhanced. Dr. Brooten further states:

> In the work that transpires between mentor and protégé, the challenge is maintaining a balance of help to further the protégé and his or her work and yet foster independence that provides the protégé with a sense of success and independence.

The protégé's success is also the mentor's success. This is sometimes difficult for some mentors to remember as the protégé becomes successful, in some instances, more successful, than the mentor. What should be a sense of pride can become a situation of conflict, particularly if the mentor's assistance is not acknowledged by the protégé. True measures of a mentor's success are the number of productive persons mentored by the mentor and later by the number of persons mentored by the mentor's original protégés—a generational phenomenon. This is a measure of external seeding and development of the discipline's next generation of researchers. This phenomenon is certainly present in the nursing discipline.

The nursing research enterprise in academe presents many challenges. The key elements in the promotion of faculty research productivity are faculty mentors who will share their expertise, time, and resources, and junior faculty who actively seek mentor relationships (Collins, 1983; Kim & Felton, 1986). In the older disciplines, senior professors are expected to facilitate the research activities of junior academics; however, this has not been the tradition in nursing. In addition, the time and resource allocation for research is frequently meager, and administrative values are not focused on this activity. Dr. Cheryl Cahill reminds us that the organizational structures and policies of many colleges and universities encourage stiff competition among faculty members for money, laboratory space, research equipment, and assistants. She states:

> It frequently appears not to be in the best interest of seasoned faculty researchers to facilitate a new colleague in the competition for limited resources. The administrator who is most successful in developing a strong and diverse research portfolio in the organization will create an atmosphere that discourages internal competition and rewards collaboration—this is not easy. Just as in some cultures, it takes a village to rear a child, the organizational culture that is most conducive to research productivity is one that recognizes that it takes the whole faculty to support a scientist. The administrator who wishes to lead an organization with a strong research focus that supports and nurtures novice researchers must create an organization that views each member as a mentor and serves as a mentoring organization. Organizational rewards should

be devised that encourage the development of mentor-protégé dyads in the research enterprise.

An area of crucial importance for the profession is enhancing the presence of nursing research activity in acute care hospitals, where 60% of the practicing nurses are employed. The key to success in conducting research in the clinical setting is the presence of mentorship. According to Lough (1986), a *networking mentor* can help the staff nurse to establish institutional contacts to facilitate the research, while a *research mentor's* contribution is to help transfer a clinical problem into a research question. Research activity can improve the image that staff nurses have of themselves as professionals. Ultimately, this form of esteem building can lead to a renewed commitment to quality, which translates into improved patient care. These were the dreams of some nurses who initiated a mentoring circle for research at Broward General Medical Center in Ft. Lauderdale, Florida (Boykin & Schoenhofer, 1993). This initiative grew out of the Nursing Research Development Network of the College of Nursing at Florida Atlantic University, which was established by Dr. Savina Schoenhofer as a support system for regional nursing services to strengthen nursing research opportunities.

A Mentoring Circle: Facilitating Nursing Research with Staff Nurses

by Savina Schoenhofer and Mariamma Pyngolil

The goal of creating a new culture for nursing service at Broward General Medical Center included nursing research as a key component of that effort. With Mariamma as the chair of the research committee and Savina serving as the faculty liaison and mentor, staff nurses and nurse managers have approved research proposals, served as a mentoring resource to nurses, integrated research utilization in nursing practice, and conducted research studies. The committee has developed tremendously in the 5 years since its inception. Now the members, who are staff nurses and nurse managers, provide consultation to other institutions as they start their research committees. This outstanding growth was made possible through strong mentoring activities that included guidance and direction, validation, constructive criticism and feedback, sharing expertise, providing moral support, and being present. Our own mentor relationship served as a role model for the entire group, and the research committee grew into a caring group whose members actively supported and mentored each other. Many committee members later shared that they came to the meetings because they felt support and encouragement and that it was a place that fostered professional and personal growth. We believe that it was the presence of mentor relationships among the members that cultivated a climate of collegiality and caring. The mentoring circle now encompasses four major fields of nursing endeavor: research, practice, education, and administration. This circle has extended beyond our own setting, and it is hoped it will make a contribution to the discipline in a larger arena. The ever-widening circle of nursing research that we influenced through our mentor relationships seems to have no boundaries. We have presented the research activities of our circle as an exemplar at state and national conferences, consulted widely, and received extramural funds for a large federal project. While these tangible outcomes of the mentoring circle are significant, intangible outcomes accruing from mentor relationships also are a deep source of satisfaction. We each value our heightened sense of self-confidence as mentors; even more, we value our staff nurse colleagues as enthusiastic, competent participants in nursing research endeavors.

In summary, it is clear that mentoring is a vital component of scholarship and research in the nursing profession (Bryne, Kangas, & Warren, 1996; Linc & Campbell, 1995; Rempusheski, 1992). It is reported that the most productive (eight or more research articles in a 3-year period) faculty members were more likely to have coauthored papers with mentors while in graduate school (Megel, Langston, & Creswell, 1988). Dr. Afaf Ibrahim Meleis believes that collaborative mentorship for scholarship and disciplinary progress is the best model. Dr. Meleis notes:

> Properties and patterns of mentorship are shaped by multiple societal and disciplinary forces, including the changing nature of scholarship (Boyer, 1990), increasing diversity, heightened consciousness about the oppressive history of women and nurses, and greater openness to alternate philosophical and methodological approaches in research and practice. If we want scholarship to represent application, clinical practice, and teaching in addition to research and discovery, then we

might consider establishing a collaborative mentorship model that presumes reciprocity and flexibility of roles and is shaped by these principles:

- Mentorship is multidimensional. Seeking different mentors for different goals is essential.
- Mentor relationships are horizontal, not paternal or maternal.
- Mentor relationships are flexible and constantly negotiable.
- Mentor relationships are empowering and include proactivism, consciousness-raising and facilitation processes.
- Powerful and goal-achieving mentor relationships are enhanced by integration with communities of scholars.

Mentors and protégés in nursing reverse accepted forms of old patterns. The nature of mentorship within the context of our discipline, the needs of society, and global issues will be based on collaboration that involves working together, sharing ideas and research, interpreting and implementing together.

9

Group and Collective Mentorship

Does mentoring have to be the ubiquitous, often isolating dyadic model that has existed since the time of Homer? My vision of the future is a collaborative, inclusive one that welcomes diversity. Our new evolving mentor relationships will be central to this vision of collaboration and community (Mary Boose Walker).

Historically, the mentor relationship was dyadic in nature, consisting of two persons. Increasingly, we are witnessing the phenomenon of collective mentoring, in which an entire organization or association, school group, or community engages in various mentoring activities. An experience of "mentoring the community" is described by Dr. Patricia Castiglia, in which health care professionals and community members served as mentors to each other. This reciprocal partnership occurred as a result of a Community Partnership Project funded by the W. K. Kellogg Foundation, which attempts to change the way health care professionals are educated to reflect a multidisciplinary, community-oriented approach (Castiglia, 1996).

Community and Health Professional Mentor Relationships

by Patricia Castiglia

In conference rooms at rural health academic centers located on the West Texas-Mexico border, health care professionals are often reminded to "get real." This is the community health worker's way of saying that a comment does not reflect the community perspective. Community members are mentoring health care professionals and their students so that they can truly understand what a community is and how to be effective there. At another site, several community health workers are participating in a seminar on family violence and learning how to make appropriate referrals. The discussion is being led by a mental health nursing faculty member and a social work faculty member. These health care professionals are mentoring community members so they can develop a professional role and responsibilities. As in all mentoring situations, there are two participants, the mentor and the protégé. Each may take on, at different points, mentoring or protégé functions. In a community situation, in the early stages of the partnering relationship, community members may need to be mentored to develop assertiveness and leadership qualities. Later, they will become the mentors in helping academics to understand the realities and subtleties of their communities. For this role reversal to be successful, an environment of trust, openness, support, and training must be created.

How can community members be reempowered and prepared to assume greater responsibility for their community's welfare? We believe that mentor relationships can assist in this, if appropriately implemented. It was clear in the El Paso project that not only those who were directly involved in the project—the health care professionals—would serve as mentors, but the community members also would mentor the professionals. It must be a reciprocal relationship. Community members are experts about their own communities, but they had to experience an environment that would allow them to see themselves in a mentoring role. That meant that we had to develop roles for them that they and the health professionals would respect and that would provide an ambience conducive to trust and the ability to mentor. Each partner—professional and community—has to let go of some roles and behaviors from the past and develop new and expanded roles and identities. There also is a value component that must be present. Each mentor, regardless of background, must feel that what she or he is doing is valued by colleagues and the community.

A combination of formal and informal mentor programs was

instituted in this project. We found that our reciprocal mentoring model is very successful. In these relationships, mutually determined goals can be reached in an efficacious manner. Durability over time is yet to be ascertained. Implementing and maintaining health care professional education in the community require a variety of strategies. It is obvious that increased educational and mentoring activities must occur in primary care and community settings since greater numbers of practitioners will be needed there.

In the world of politics, the "old boys' network" consisted of mentoring components. Gaining entrée into the political arena required the mentorship of party leaders, who would serve as advocates and sponsors, open political doors, and assist in fund-raising. The following story describes political mentoring, a form of collective mentorship that occurred in a fledgling political action committee for nurses.

The Good Ol' Girls and Collective Mentoring

by Judith Kline Leavitt and Diana J. Mason

New York State Nurses for Political Action (NYS-NPA) was formed in the late '70s by a small group of risk-taking women in nursing who were activists on behalf of organizing nurses for political involvement. For over 15 years, it was the only political action committee for nurses in New York State. This group paved the way for successive generations of nurse activists, many of whom went on to leadership positions in various professional, policy, and political circles. Bringing in new members to this volunteer organization meant that we had to strengthen their commitment to political activism through our personal mentorship. The same process that we had established among ourselves that made us feel cared about and mentored as we learned about political organizing, fund-raising, and public speaking was what we in turn provided to newcomers to the group. By giving responsibility to novices, we believed we demonstrated our faith in their ability to learn—as long as we made ourselves available to mentor each one. Our mentoring activities included:

- networking that extended to nurses, students, and politicians;

- providing information about and assistance with career opportunities;
- sponsoring individuals for political skills workshops;
- creating new titles and positions in response to innovative ideas and rewarding individual commitment;
- developing personal friendships from a shared commitment to the mission of the group;
- developing skills in public speaking;
- taking novices on lobbying visits to policy makers;
- sharing political strategies for influencing policy makers;
- participating in constructive critiques of new experiences with policy makers and political campaigns; and
- accepting newcomers as full members with an equal voice and vote and recommending them for increasingly responsible positions.

In analyzing the ingredients of the successful group mentorship that occurred, we identified the following principles:

- A collective vision and commitment must override individual ambition.
- Sharing the mentoring of newcomers by the whole group enables the newcomers to benefit from the different strengths of mentors. The shared sense of responsibility also prevents the newcomers from becoming too dependent on any individual and encourages greater independence.
- A feminist context that embraces a collective, nonhierarchical approach shaped the vision and the process for the group.
- The norm of power sharing often coexisted with a healthy competitive spirit because the competition centered on ideas rather than people.
- Valuing diverse ideas and viewpoints encourages the group to acknowledge and support a newcomer's strengths and contributions, as well as share responsibilities for running an organization.
- A sense of caring was conveyed and extended to each of us as multidimensional people. This personal involvement fostered a collective commitment to each

person and created a sense of belonging and caring that was important to us as nurses.

If this sounds too good to be true, let us assure you that there are always difficult times within organizations that exist purely by volunteer effort and with limited financial resources. When we had challenging times, it was usually because the chairperson and members, due to time and distance, were unable to mentor and nurture the collective spirit. This became critical as board membership became statewide rather than remaining at the local level. In recounting the influence of NYS-NPA on our lives, we have found ourselves trying to recreate collective mentoring in other professional situations. We discovered that this kind of support is not always easy to find. We are convinced, however, that collective mentoring is a value about process and working together to extend nursing's solidarity of activists. It also is about recognizing that new, even inexperienced, voices can contribute to the development of the most seasoned mentors. Finally, collective mentoring is about moving a vision in creative ways and being committed to the development of people who can move that vision. We are all winners when we can mentor in collective ways, learn together, care for each other and our achievements, and celebrate together.

Leadership development also is being fostered by collective mentoring in various organizations and associations. A survey conducted by the American College of Healthcare Executives (ACHE) found that while women, including nurses, are poised to assume significant leadership roles within hospitals, important collective changes must be made for them to advance into these leadership roles. The ACHE has issued a policy statement, "Responsibility for Mentoring," that encourages its 30,000 members to mentor early careerists and those in mid-career. ACHE's health care executive career resources center is assisting its constituents nationwide to develop formal mentoring programs and to disseminate the value of leaders mentoring others as part of their inherent responsibility (Lutz, 1995). The American Association of Colleges of Nursing (AACN), with a membership of 510 baccalaureate, master's, and doctoral nursing programs in the United States, has a strategic goal of developing academic leaders. To that end, an Executive Development Program was begun in 1989 that focused on organizational assessment and executive role development. A formal mentor component was built into this program.

Executive Development and Mentorship

by Rachel Z. Booth, Geraldine (Polly) Bednash, and Michelle F. Pratt

Persons new to the role of academic executive are provided the opportunity to engage in a 1-year mentorship with experienced American Association of Colleges of Nursing member deans. Expected outcomes include introduction and sponsorship to AACN, socialization to the dean's role, leadership development, and networking opportunities. Persons are either matched to a dean who is interested and willing to be a mentor or they have the option to choose a mentor on their own. Time, distance, and personal style have consistently been the areas of greatest difficulty for both mentors and new deans. In addition, budget constraints prevented some participants from scheduling personal meetings or attending AACN meetings to develop their relationship. The most popular forms of contact have been meetings, telephone conversations, written correspondence, and electronic mail. The top three identified issues for exploration in the mentor relationship have been the faculty, administration, and the dean's role. Other topics are budget, accreditation, program, strategic planning, evaluation, and organizational insight. Participants also reported appreciation for the opportunity to share experiences, form new relationships, learn about other institutions, gain wisdom about organizational dynamics, and try out suggestions and information about the dean's role.

An important issue for the success of the program was its structure. Some respondents reported that the idea of a "program" was misleading because it was very informally structured. It was suggested that mentors and protégés be required to contract for specific outcomes and to provide progress reports on the relationship. Others appreciate the freedom to explore issues without feeling that there are requirements to fulfill. Still others believe that a mentor relationship cannot be regulated and that "people find their own mentors." In some dyads, both new deans and mentor deans expressed frustration with each other over apparent disinterest or lack of commitment to the relationship. Many have commented that one cannot be "forced" into a mentor relationship and that mutual interest is the only way to make it a productive experience. The experience of mentoring is not neutral. In fact, it requires participants to test preconceived ideas about roles, to share sensitive information, and to provide and receive critical analysis. Reaction to this program has been generally positive. New deans have reported that the support, advice, and introductory experience far outweigh any difficulties. Mentor deans expressed gratitude for helping them to recall the fears of being a new dean and lending the benefit of their experience to a new dean. We believe that the mentor connection enhances the leadership skills of our members and provides for the development of academic leaders in nursing.

Nursing deans also engage in mentoring each other through state, regional, and special interest associations. One of these, the Association of Jesuit Colleges and Universities Conference of Nursing Programs, was established more than 20 years ago to mentor and support each other in key areas, such as curriculum, faculty exchanges, budget, and the role of nursing and nursing leadership in Jesuit colleges and universities. Dr. Cynthia Zane states that this group of 19 deans has provided strong collective and individual mentoring experiences for each other.

> There is an intrinsic cohesion with the group evolving from the common mission that supports frequent interactions and mentoring relationships among each other. We call, fax, or e-mail each other on a variety of issues. A mentoring system for deans as suggested by Vigen (1992) provides a dynamism that changes organizational life. For those of us who have had the privilege of membership in this Association, our mentorship among each other has contributed significantly to our leadership success.

Collective mentoring can also influence an entire regional program. An example of this is a report from the Southern Council on Collegiate Education for Nursing.

Creating a Legacy of Leadership in the South

by Jean A. Kelley and Eula Aiken

A 3-year grant from the Division of Nursing, U.S. Department of Health and Human Services, was awarded to the Southern

Council on Collegiate Education for Nursing (SCCEN) in 1992 to enhance graduate nursing education in the South. One of the grant elements was the development of a regional mentor program for graduate faculty and graduate program directors. The program goals were to: (a) develop aspiring, novice, and seasoned graduate nurse educators in the tripartite faculty role; (b) develop both aspiring graduate program directors and those already in the role; and (c) develop and evaluate a regional mentor program for graduate faculty and program directors. Thirty mentors and 24 protégés were participants. We devised a guide to assist the mentors and protégés that was extracted from the literature (Arnoldussen & White, 1990; Brito, 1992; Sandler, 1993; Strachura & Hoff, 1990):

THE TEN COMMANDMENTS OF MENTORING

1. Do not be afraid to mentor.
2. Do not try to fulfill or expect to have fulfilled every function of mentoring.
3. Have planned goals and expectations for communication and negotiation.
4. Inform your protégé or mentor if the mentorship is taking too much or too little time, or is not challenging.
5. Critique and be open to a critique of performance that contains praise and constructive suggestions for improvement.
6. Market the protégé's accomplishments and the mentor's support.
7. Involve the protégé or mentor in informal activities, e.g., luncheons and discussions.
8. Encourage the protégé to seek additional resources for career development, for example, financial support to attend professional meetings or to fund research projects.
9. Develop mentoring programs at state and organizational levels.
10. Be willing to mentor individuals of diverse backgrounds.

The post-3-year evaluation survey of mentors and protégés revealed that the most beneficial aspects of the program were networking, exchange of ideas, and exposure to new resources. Other reported benefits included collegial support, problem solving, career development, exploration of graduate nursing issues, strategizing, grantsmanship, and potential publications. Four stages of a full professional career described by McBride (1994) provide a blueprint for the type of nursing leader that we hope to develop through the SCCEN:

Stage 1: Protégé achieves professional competence as an academic or educational administrator.

Stage 2: Protégé makes scholarly contributions to the profession (publications, presentations, competitive grants).

Stage 3: Protégé assumes increased responsibility for mentoring others.

Stage 4: Both protégé and mentor use expertise as humanistic, problem-solving visionaries to shape the future of nursing and health care.

It will take longer than 3 years of a federal grant to create a legacy of leadership in graduate nursing education in the South. However, the commitment of the mentors and protégés to the goals of the mentor program has made it possible to launch a cadre of "influentials" in nursing education who will have a long-term effect on nursing and health care well into the 21st century.

American foundations also are investing in the development of leaders through mentoring. In 1991, the Pew Charitable Trusts Foundation initiated a Leadership Diversity Fellowship Program with the Association of Academic Health Centers in the United States. This program was designed to identify women and under-represented minorities for senior leadership positions in academic health centers and to encourage the future expression of pluralistic societal values in the health centers. It was recognized that in the 20th century there had been only four female deans of medicine and no CEO of an academic health center who was female or a member of an ethnic minority group, and that this imbalance should be addressed. One of the unique aspects of the program was the creation of a framework in which mentor relationships would develop.

Dr. Elaine Larson and Dr. Dorothy Powell, who were Scholars in the program, describe some of their experiences:

> We were assigned mentors with the expectation that we would find at least one or two persons with whom rapport and a relationship would be developed in which counseling, advice, and assistance with career advancement and professional development would occur. Scholar-protégés' experiences were varied, depending upon their career stage, their willingness to commit the time and energy necessary to establish links and to participate in the available opportunities, as well as whom they selected as mentors. From this program we learned that while you cannot mandate a mentor relationship, you can set up an atmosphere and culture in which such relationships are likely (or not) to flourish. Our mentor experiences are best described as journeys during which conflicting emotions of excitement and anxiety were present. We learned that comfort, rapport, and acceptance of the protégé as a worthy person is a critical first step in establishing the mentor relationship. The next requirement is determining what one hopes to get out of the experience and how it might enhance some personal attributes. Another principle is that mentor relationships can only develop in a milieu of safe, honest disclosure. After exploring professional goals and needs, arriving at clear goals for the mentoring experience provided a road map for potential learning. The final empowering lesson of mentorship is the realization that you have a lifelong advocate and friend who has a vested interest in you. Our membership in the Fellowship Program continues to influence us. Through our mentor connections, we have experienced a broadening of our worlds, a heightened self-confidence, and possession of the potential for new or altered life directions. We feel very fortunate for the influence of our mentors in this special leadership development opportunity.

PART V

Expanding the Mentor Connection

10

Global and Cross-Cultural Mentoring: Voices from the Field

> The culture of caring that is uniquely nursing can act as a mutual language for mentorship across cultures (Gioiella, Natapoff, & McDermott).

Mentor connections are increasingly occurring in a global context. These cross-cultural relationships are characterized by a diversity of partnerships and collaborative linkages. This collaboration occurs among nurses, teachers, students, and consumers of nursing care. International mentoring is manifested by a true mutuality of sharing and a reciprocity of giving and receiving. Partners in these relationships are challenged by communication, distance, cultural and language differences, and economics. Whether one mentors in one's own country, but within a specific cultural context, or in a different country, it requires trust, openness, flexibility, and sensitivity. The International Association for Mentoring was founded in 1986 out of a vision to bring together diverse groups from all sectors internationally, including education, health and human services, business, government, and community-based organizations. The association supports and promotes global mentoring through public forums, developmental activities, and the dissemination of materials on research and models of effective mentoring.

Cross-cultural collaborative mentoring calls for pioneers and change agents who are willing to engage in the unknown and the sometimes uncomfortable. By its very nature, this mentorship generates synergy and empowerment that come with forging new models and patterns of working and living. The culture of nursing, with its value and perspective of caring, provides a framework of unity amid diversity. The sisterhood and brotherhood of nursing allows an easy acceptance of differences and the recognition of the importance of sharing. Therefore, there is unprecedented opportunity for creating professional and social change through cross-cultural mentoring that provides transformation in perspectives, knowledge, skills, and attitudes (Morales-Mann & Higuchi, 1995). This fundamental change can begin with a kernel of the mentor relationship among colleagues that subsequently influences an entire organization or school, the profession, and the larger environment. Mentorship is a powerful mechanism for driving change across global boundaries.

The nursing profession has developed an impressive track record of global collaboration and mentorship. Nurses are venturing into cyberspace and communicating around the world with their colleagues. The narratives in this chapter illustrate the various dimensions of nurses' mentorship with each other. These span professional and program development, research, practice, and leadership and career development. Through these stories shine the beauty and power of the diversity and the unity of our mentor relationships on behalf of nursing's work.

Mentoring for International Educational Program Development

by Joyce J. Fitzpatrick

The classic mentor-protégé relationship, in which the mentor is an older, more experienced person who guides and nurtures a younger, less experienced colleague (Vance & Olson, 1991), supports the basic understanding for this story, while recognizing that the person being mentored often provides substantial learning for the mentor. This is especially true in international relationships because the learning that occurs is most often mutually beneficial. Highly effective international relationships are in fact characterized by *partnerships*. Within these relationships, it is possible to discern many types of mentoring, in which both parties mutually progress in their career development and role socialization. Various types of mentor relationships can exist among international colleagues. These include mentoring with international students, mentoring among exchange students and faculty, and mentor relationships among international colleagues. The mentor relationship is a partnership. Mentoring among international colleagues approaches a full partnership, with mutually beneficial outcomes.

MENTORING OF INTERNATIONAL STUDENTS

While my experience with mentoring international students is with graduate students who come to the United States to obtain postbasic preparation, the same principles apply to all levels of students. One important factor is that international students often are already in leadership positions in nursing education or health care in their own countries. They have been selected through a rigorous review process and are being supported by their governments personally and financially to pursue graduate education. They are usually guaranteed key leadership positions upon return to their countries. Against this background, it is important that they are mentored successfully and that the student-protégés and their mentors understand and discuss the roles for which the students are being prepared. Faculty mentors in the host country must be cognizant of the health care and nursing education systems that the students will enter once they return to their home countries. It is most helpful if the mentor can visit the sponsoring country to obtain a firsthand view of the political and environmental realities and to make an assessment of the strengths and limitations of the situation. If the mentor has international experience in the student's country and is familiar with the culture, the mentor relationship will be enhanced.

One important challenge of the international mentor relationship is to continue the partnership once the student has assumed a leadership position in his or her home country. This continued contact is particularly important in developing worldwide relationships in nursing. Through such relationships, faculty can facilitate cross-cultural research. An example of a planned approach to continued mentor relationships and the building of a team approach to cross-cultural research is a collaborative breast cancer project undertaken by a team of faculty, international Ph.D. graduates, and students at Case Western Reserve University. The original idea for the collaborative cross-cultural research project arose when the faculty mentor discovered that two international students had similar research interests. One student was studying psychological responses to the life-threatening experience of women newly diagnosed with breast cancer, and the other student was exploring the psychological and personal meanings of health and illness. The plan for a collaborative project was initiated as the students worked together to find a common conceptual and empirical ground, preserving the uniqueness of each student's dissertation research. Two additional faculty mentors joined the project, adding the potential of having more countries represented in this cross-cultural research project. Additional team members have been added from the international student group, who will carry out the project in their countries as part of a thesis or dissertation, pooling the data for comparative analyses. This example could be multiplied with careful planning among faculty mentors and international graduate students.

Another important feature of the faculty mentor-international student relationship is the development of opportunities for coauthored publications and presentations. Often, the publication arena provides avenues for a reciprocal partnership. For example, the faculty mentor is often asked to publish in journals and newsletters of the countries sponsoring the students. Following a consultation trip to Taiwan, I was asked if two presentations could be translated into Chinese (by the students) so that they could be disseminated more widely in the country. Faculty mentors of international students should develop joint publications and scholarly presentations.

MENTOR RELATIONSHIPS AMONG EXCHANGE STUDENTS
AND FACULTY

The reciprocal partnership model is even more evident among students and faculty who formally exchange positions with each other, even for a limited period of time. During this time, these individuals also exchange mentors. It is very helpful to the individual to know ahead of time whom they can count on in the new situation and country to provide mentoring. In fact, delineation of the professional mentor relationships can be a formal part of the proposed contractual relationship between the two sponsoring institutions. If not a formal part of the relationship, exploration of the possible mentors before the exchange is initiated would be beneficial. If there is no formal provision for mentors in the host institution, the exchange student or faculty member should inquire about this from the sponsoring institution or host. For example, many of our international visiting faculty and students request specific information about faculty who might be conducting research in the international visitors' areas of expertise. Therefore, in arranging the visit it becomes very important to schedule meetings with key faculty mentors and experts in the designated areas.

Mentor Relationships among International Colleagues

This third type of mentoring—among international colleagues—most closely resembles a true mutual partnership, where each member understands that he or she receives as much guidance in role socialization and career development as he or she gives to colleagues. While career development may be along different dimensions, it is an important component of a full partnership that the learning and exchange be mutually beneficial. For example, one colleague may develop skills in formal scientific presentations and the other may develop skills in political presentations to a government agency. An international colleague who has experience with multiple languages may help to clarify conceptualizations and thus add to their precision. In developing international relationships, in particular those with mentoring characteristics, it is important for both parties to possess some understanding of each other's culture and language.

Summary

With the advent of technology, global communication has been enhanced and travel has been facilitated. International projects and relationships within nursing education and practice have been extended. Concomitant with the future increase in international projects, conferences and cross-cultural research will be an increasing demand for stronger, global mentor relationships.

Global Mentoring: A Collaborative Process

by Carol Picard

For several years, I have been involved in a collaborative mentoring relationship with Dr. Galina Perfiljeva, dean of the School of Nursing at the I. M. Sechenov Moscow Medical Academy in Russia. This experience has taught me a great deal about what mentoring can be on a global basis. What is different about this kind of mentoring? Frequently, there is no age difference between the persons in the relationship. The knowledge and information that is shared is more a function of each person's access to what is unique in her country and not a difference in level of expertise. We are both experts in our own areas. We have areas where our knowledge overlaps and areas where we can learn a great deal from each other. We mentor each other. I needed a mentor to help me understand nursing in Russia. Galina needed a mentor to help her gain access to resources and nurse leaders in the United States. That is our fit.

In developing global mentoring relationships, it is important to hear the call of one's colleague. Much like responding to our patients' needs, it is critical that we listen to what is needed in the mentoring relationship and not what we think is needed. It is important to invite and honor the requests. Let me illustrate. In 1990, when nurses began to travel more frequently between Russia and the United States, everything that Western nurses brought or shared was received enthusiastically. Now, as Russian nurses reflect on what is needed in their country, they are more selective and look for how Western resources will fit into their own health care system. An example is hospice. The volunteer projects in our hospice programs were greeted with enthusiasm and incorporated into one of the first Russian hospices by Kira Apraksina, nursing director. The concepts of self-care and empowerment are not as well received. The role of the patient and the Russian conception of suffering as a part of life to be endured interfere with some strategies suggested by American nurses.

Much like a good consultant, we must wait for the request, all the while learning. The World Health Organization has materials on nursing and health care in countries worldwide which give some perspective on what the situation of nurses is in a particular country. My readings on Russia have been not only in health care, but in history, politics, culture, literature and social issues. What my Russian colleagues have to teach me is about a rich heritage and how to be extraordinarily creative with limited resources. I also need to understand before I attempt to act. It is a fair assumption to say that most other countries know more about the United States than we know about them. Learning at least rudiments of the foreign language where one is working is important to that nursing community as well.

In our relationship, Galina and I have identified certain areas on which to focus. The first is people and communications. Since our relationship began, Galina has visited the United States several times, presenting papers on those occasions. My work has been to identify conferences where she might present, submitting joint abstracts, and getting information about programs to her. On each trip, I have made arrangements for her to meet nurse leaders and to seek their help in getting materials to her once she returned to Russia. On each of my trips to her country, she has provided the same support. Our overall focus is education, since we are both academics. I have worked to get textbooks and journal materials for her students and faculty. In collaboration with nonnursing faculty at Fitchburg State College, we are responding to Galina's call for an English as a Second Language (ESL) text using nursing materials for her graduate students. We also have published two papers and presented two symposia together. Galina has begun the first nursing research journal in her country. She has asked for assistance in selecting articles from American nursing journals from which she might get copyright permission to translate into Russian. I look for the help of other nurse scholars to assist me with this project. The issue of financial support for projects became critical as we explored how to publish the ESL text, how to encourage young nurse scholars from her graduate program to come to the United States, and how to support her program with some technology. A friend of Russian nursing, businessman Sean McGivern offered to make available Russian lacquer pins as a fund-raising item to Fitchburg State College's chapter of Sigma Theta Tau International, of which Galina is a member. In an 8-month period, with the support of an enthusiastic membership, we raised over $17,000 for our Russian nursing project. Our chapter has also taken a group of American nurse leaders to Russia and is planning other trips. We were able to celebrate the first graduation of master's-prepared nurses in Russia's history at Galina's academy in June 1995. Knowing how important and historical this event was, I gathered letters of congratulations into a booklet, including greetings from Vice President Albert Gore, other political leaders and nurse leaders in practice, education, and research. Galina was delighted to share this booklet with the rector of her academy and many colleagues and friends.

There are challenges in global mentor relationships. To link our two worlds, it helped to have a belief in the impossible. Our biggest challenge is communication. The mail in Russia is notoriously slow, and telephone contact is expensive. Electronic mail works some of the time, depending on the telephone lines, and so patience is a premium virtue. We have as an important resource a colleague-friend (Mr. McGivern) who travels to Russia regularly and hand-carries materials back and forth. This is a commitment to maintaining our relationship over time. Galina and I know each other better now than in 1990 and have a richer picture of each other's experiences and resources. Our goals for the future are to mentor clinical nurses and nurse researchers in clinical demonstration projects and to link American and Russian nurses in clinical agencies and colleges via the Internet. We are bridge builders. Our collaborative mentoring relationship has been very exciting for me, both personally and professionally. Galina always ends her presentations with the thought that nursing has no borders. As nurses, we all have the same goal of health and comfort for patients, wherever in the world they may be. Global mentoring can help us achieve this goal.

The Hunter–Shanghai Project: An International Cross-Cultural Experience in Research Mentorship

by Evelynn C. Gioiella, Janet N. Natapoff, and Mary Anne N. McDermott

SETTING THE STAGE

In the late 1980s, Hunter-Bellevue School of Nursing in New York received a letter from Lu Tanyun in which she described herself as a teacher of nursing in the Department of Nursing at Shanghai Medical University (SMU), the People's Republic of China, requesting the opportunity to come to Hunter-Bellevue as a visiting scholar for 6 months. Her goal was to learn about baccalaureate education in the United States. This letter set into motion a mentoring experience among several nursing faculty and some 30 Chinese nurses. This mentorship, which began with a focus on nursing education, evolved into collaborative nursing research, which expanded to include multiple sites on four continents—North America, Europe, Asia, and Africa. This story recounts the development of the Hunter-Shanghai Project, with the successes and difficulties that have accompanied its growth.

Our goal in arranging for Ms. Lu's visit was to facilitate the development of baccalaureate nursing education in China, also the goal of SMU. The first difficulty with the proposed experience became apparent the evening Ms. Lu arrived from China. Dean Gioiella and Professor Natapoff met Ms. Lu for a welcoming dinner. Ms. Lu had written letters in excellent English and had described her spoken English as very good. This was not the case. Ms. Lu's English reading skills were good; however, her comprehension skills were just adequate, and her verbal skills in English made communication a struggle. Communication competency has been an ongoing hurdle for all of us involved in the Hunter-Shanghai Project and is a key element in any international mentoring experience. Ms. Lu worked intensively on her English and with several nursing faculty. By the end of the semester she had learned a significant amount about the nursing program and, most important, had established a close relationship with one faculty member who became her personal mentor.

The next phase of the Hunter-Shanghai Project began with an invitation from SMU for Dean Gioiella to visit to "lay a foundation for further exchanges between our two schools of nursing." Expenses for the visit were to be paid by SMU. The letter explained that the Department of Nursing had become a School of Nursing, the first in China, and was interested in more "academic exchanges." Dean Gioiella was named a visiting professor, asked to give several lectures, and to address the possibility of research cooperation in the future. Clearly, the goals that SMU had for the academic exchange had expanded and changed focus. Dean Gioiella was now being asked to facilitate nursing research at SMU. The visit resulted in an agreement between Hunter-Bellevue School of Nursing and SMU School of Nursing to explore opportunities for joint nursing research. The research projects would be conducted by two professors from Hunter, using coinvestigators from SMU. The Hunter faculty would serve as mentors for the coinvestigators, and the studies would be conducted in Shanghai. SMU had funds to support the faculty visitors for a week if Hunter provided travel costs. Since the goals for Hunter had now shifted to facilitating faculty research, funds available for this purpose were allocated. Two professors, Dr. Janet Natapoff and Dr. Mary Anne McDermott, who had previous experience in China and cross-cultural research, undertook the next phase of the mentorship. The purpose of the Hunter-Shanghai Research Project, as it had now evolved, was to teach the research process through active participation in ongoing research studies. A secondary purpose was to help our Chinese colleagues develop a program of research that was appropriate for their setting. This kind of exchange involves more than teaching through a series of lectures. The traditional visiting scholar usually gives lectures in English with a translator at hand. Instead, this project involved real mentoring—intense, sustained interactions on the part of both parties, much support, and emotional investment.

THE JOURNEY

Abstracts of proposals for three possible research studies were sent to Dean Yang Yinhua, at the SMU School of Nursing in Shanghai, by Professors Natapoff and McDermott. Two of the proposals were extensions of ongoing quantitative research projects with American samples, and the third was an original qualitative descriptive proposal to look at perceptions of pain. The Hunter researchers were notified that the three proposals were accepted enthusiastically as vehicles for learning research "by doing." Meanwhile, under the leadership of Dean Yang, three research teams composed of nurse faculty specialists and clinical nursing leaders were established in Shanghai. The leader of each team was a faculty member who spoke English. These leaders became coinvestigators and, because we spent the most time with them, our "protégés."

The day after arriving in Shanghai, Natapoff and McDermott met with each research team to answer questions and negotiate the final methodologies for each study. Since China and the United States have such different cultures, values, and beliefs, all three studies had to be adapted to China, while still ultimately allowing for researchers to compare Chinese and American data. As mentors, care had to be taken to avoid inadvertently forcing American ideas on the protégés. As researchers, commitment to the research process during the learning experience was paramount. Guidance, support, and negotiation, all responsibilities of a mentor, were evidenced during the bicultural research team interactions. However, since faculty members are colleagues, both Chinese and American researchers felt a sense of ownership and responsibility for the studies. By the 2nd day, after very intensive work, the teams were collecting data. By the 5th day, preliminary data for each study were analyzed. During those 5 days, Natapoff and McDermott worked with the teams and team leaders for many hours. The growing reality of our mutual research goals served as impetus and energy for the long hours involved in the initiation of the three projects. While the Hunter researchers wanted the project to be a success because it would extend original studies into cross-cultural research, the idea of advancing the research knowledge base among Chinese nurse colleagues was the driving force. As part of the project, we also had to work out ownership of the research. All agreed that the Chinese data would be published in China, with the research team leaders as senior authors. To date, one study has been published and two have been submitted for publication. When Chinese data are reported as part of cross-cultural studies, they will be published in international journals with the American principal investigators as first authors and the Chinese coinvestigators as second authors.

Many of the difficulties of working with colleagues in the same university occur when working with those from other countries, but are compounded by geographical distance, language, and cultural differences. For example, people in different cultures work at different paces and have different ideas on how to interpret data. Consensus is hard to achieve even when researchers know each other well. Despite what seems to be complete agreement on methodology, people still go out and do what they think is best. Thus it is with international research. Some of these difficulties were as apparent with the China project as they are with any research, but were compounded by the mentorship arrangement. One of the purposes of the project was to help Chinese faculty develop a program of research. They were student protégés in the project at the same time they were being encouraged to become independent. One group added a subset to their sample because the population was available and interesting. Another submitted an article for publication before the final data analysis was completed. Without direct supervision, it is impossible to monitor data collection. This is true even when data collectors and researchers live in the same city. Despite complications, the project was amazingly successful. The Chinese faculty members remained enthusiastic, very interested in research and in the research process, energetic, capable, and, perhaps most important, continued to learn from the transcultural mentoring relationship. Within 3 months, more than 500 subjects had been interviewed for the two quantitative studies. The data were coded and readied for analysis. Data were also collected from 15 subjects for the pilot phase of the third study. Another visit was made 18 months after the initial visit. All three studies were reviewed by the individual teams and their leaders. Results of data analysis done in New York were shared with the group. Plans to begin the second phase of the qualitative study on pain were finalized. This visit served to reinforce the mentoring experience and to "launch" the Chinese nurses into independent work.

Issues in Cross-Cultural Mentoring

Mentoring is usually defined as "a close relationship between two people that takes place over a period of time." The mentor is committed to developing the protégé and facilitating opportunities for advancement. This is difficult to do when the two parties are separated by thousands of miles, come from very different cultures, and speak different languages. Yet such differences can be bridged. The mutual desire to teach about and use research as a basis for practice forms a common bond for nurses across continents. The culture of caring that is uniquely nursing can act as a mutual language for mentorship across cultures. Acknowledging the difficulties, while drawing energy from the similarities, can support future cross-cultural mentoring in nursing. It is essential that the mentor have at least some knowledge of the protégé's culture and is comfortable in settings that are different from home. A tangible outcome or product of the initial mentoring experience, such as a completed research project, will provide evidence to the protégés of the professional value of the relationship. The Hunter-Shanghai Project had such a product: two completed research studies and one still in progress.

"Learning by doing" was another technique that enhanced success for the project. The protégés, Chinese research teams and leaders, were involved in the selection of the research studies, had input into methodologies, and performed initial data collection under the direct guidance of the mentors. The protégés were able to immediately see the results of their labor. At the same time, because of immediate direct feedback from the mentors, they could feel secure in their newly learned research activities. This is probably one of the major reasons why the project was successful. It would have been simpler and less physically and emotionally draining if the mentors had lectured about the research process, told the protégés how to do the research after their departure, and simply asked for a written progress report. The "hands-off" approach requires far less direct guidance, and the relationship is certainly less intense. However, the hands-off approach would not be authentic mentoring, and it would be more difficult to control for the effects of culture for cross-cultural comparisons. There also would be the lost opportunity for direct feedback and necessary encouragement for the novice researchers.

There is another very practical issue related to global mentoring endeavors. Although financial support for any study is a concern, the problems escalate with international research because of the high costs of travel and communication. Visits to a foreign country often are the responsibility of the mentor. Foreign nurses, especially those from Third World countries, do not have access to the funds necessary for travel. Since nursing education is frequently not a national priority for underdeveloped countries, government support is often lacking and private funds are nonexistent. From a research perspective, it is probably more effective for American mentors to travel to the place where the research learning and activity is to occur. Novice researchers, even if it were possible for them to travel to America, might not be able to translate newly learned research techniques into activities when they return to their own environment. Culturally related problem solving can be accomplished when the mentor and protégé have discussions in the environment of the new research. Support for expensive travel abroad, even when research related, is becoming harder to find because of budget constraints.

Less obvious is the cost of communication, which can be prohib-itive unless carefully planned. Direct airmail is costly but man-ageable. To reduce mail costs, Chinese researchers were taught to code data on code sheets prior to the mentors' departure. When only code sheets, and not original data, are mailed, costs are kept to a minimum. If computers and FAX machines are available in the foreign country, data can be transported via FAX, thus saving both time and money. Once data are received, the cost of data analysis must be negotiated. For the Hunter-Shanghai Project, a small university grant funded the analysis phase of the quantita-tive studies.

Toward the Future

All things new—whether experiences of learning, doing, or just being in a different place than before—frequently evoke feelings of insecurity and sometimes cause us to retreat to activities and places that are more familiar. Nursing in the United States and other industrial countries has grown and flourished because of the willingness of nurses to be adventuresome and experiment with new ways of mentoring and new ways of thinking. American nurses have led foreign colleagues in the idea of research-based clinical practice. We have aroused the curiosity and motivation of colleagues around the world to emulate our mentoring experiences. American nurse researchers will con-tinue to be approached by nurses in foreign countries who desire to learn about research and who understand the need to develop their own culturally appropriate research-based practice. The initial request from a Chinese nurse to learn about American baccalaureate nursing education led to an awareness of the value of research-based practice. Dean Gioiella's first response was that a way had to be found to support the professional dreams of our Shanghai colleagues. Professors Natapoff and McDermott overcame their initial anxiety about trying new teaching-learn-ing strategies in a different environment. The knowledge that they could meet a probable mentoring criterion of "ability to think on one's feet" helped them to put insecurity aside and ini-tiate a new type of teaching-learning mentor-protégé relation-ship. Upon reflection, faculty of the Hunter-Bellevue School of Nursing have gained far more than they gave. Just as a mentor-ing experience in research was given to our Shanghai nursing colleagues, they unknowingly provided us with mentoring in cross-cultural caring.

The New Zealand Midwifery Mentor Partnership

by Karen Guilliland

The woman and midwife mentor partnership is the foundation on which the midwifery profession and its practitioners have developed in New Zealand during the last decade. This relationship between women and midwives working together toward a shared goal achieved radical change within the maternity services throughout the country. Women mentored midwives to reach their potential as autonomous practitioners by believing in them and demanding an alternative to the medical model of care in childbirth. Midwives responded with a confidence that comes from a supportive society and a raised awareness of their own abilities and pressed for the right to offer services independent from the medical profession.

This mentoring partnership between women and midwives culminated in legislative change in 1990, giving midwives the ability to practice autonomously. They were given statutory equivalence with the medical practitioners and charged with providing the primary health maternity service. This legislative mandate included diagnosis and investigation, hospital admitting privileges, prescribing and treatment abilities, and equal pay (Department of Health, 1990). As with all successful mentoring relationships, the benefits for both partners—women and midwives—have been empowering and reciprocal. The effects of this process have been comprehensive and way beyond the original expectations of those involved. As a result of our mentoring and partnering in every aspect of the childbearing experience (political, professional, and personal), midwives and women are deconstructing the medical model of childbirth toward a midwifery model, redefining professionalism, changing societal attitudes and expectations about women and childbirth, and thereby increasing women's self-determination and control of their own experiences (Tully, 1994). The uniqueness of this model is that it is women led. It is present not only between client and midwife but midwife and consumer group, midwife and doctor, midwife and professional organization, and teacher and student. The partnership can be defined as a relationship of "sharing between the woman and midwife, involving trust, shared control, responsibility and shared meaning through mutual understanding" (Guilliland & Pairman, 1995). The story of how changes to the maternity service and midwifery autonomy were achieved demonstrates clearly the value of partnership and offers a working model of mentoring in action.

The development of midwifery in a mentoring framework reflects a distinctly New Zealand pattern of living. In a small, relatively egalitarian, bicultural society, it is possible to easily experience mentoring, networking, and sharing of knowledge. It is the bicultural nature of New Zealand that has exposed its people to a different way of viewing their world. The constitutional and legislative structure of New Zealand society is founded on the Treaty of Waitangi, which identifies three principles that govern the relationship between Maori (the indigenous people) and the Crown. These principles are partnership, participation, and protection. New Zealand society's exposure to the rights and responsibilities inherent in honoring these principles has facilitated women's understanding of midwifery as a partnership. The common feature of Maori claims for sovereignty and women's demand for control over their childbearing experience is the rejection by both of their oppression by the dominant cultures of *Pakeha* (European) and medicine. Women in New Zealand in the 1950s were demanding changes in the maternity service, but midwives did not join forces with women until the mid-1980s. The impetus for midwives was their realization that medicine and nursing had almost entirely subsumed midwifery from its autonomous base into a branch of nursing dependent on medicine (Donley, 1986). Legislative and educational changes further eroded the midwife's role. Midwifery's most significant political action was to acknowledge this loss of its identity and knowledge base and join forces with women to reclaim jurisdiction over childbirth. The midwives formed their own separate body in 1989 to legitimate their professional independence. The establishment of the New Zealand College of Midwives included equal membership for the women and consumer groups who had mentored the midwifery profession to this point. Midwives recognized their obligation to women and that their status as a profession was reliant on honoring and maintaining the social mandate women had given to them (Rothman, 1984). The professional body for midwives was, therefore, established in partnership with women and various consumer groups. It was the influence and strength of this political partnership that then flowed into the midwife and woman relationship. After 1990, midwives deserted the fragmentation of the hospital-based system to work independently from a community base, and women welcomed the service with open arms. Continuity of care enabled the midwife and the woman to form a relationship that could make a difference in the medical power base predominant in New Zealand and in most Western childbirth services.

Several events allowed this to happen. Midwives had a major mind shift to believe that their allegiances and professional base must lie with women, not the health organizations or employers. Women mentored and lobbied for midwives to attend them. Given that strength to initiate independent practice, midwives were affirmed further and encouraged by the mentoring partnership they built with their clients. The reciprocity of this partnership was clearly felt by both the midwife and her clients. When a relationship is mutually beneficial, both partners are empowered. Midwives and women discussed and refined their expectations of each other and continue to do so. The way in which this relationship flourishes is no different than in any other successful mentor relationship. Each partner is valued as bringing knowledge, skills, and experience. The relationship is dynamic and negotiated individually. Responsibility and power are shared, with the aim of increasing women's control over their experiences. The woman decides the importance of others within this partnership, and the midwife facilitates the family's knowledge and understanding. As with all relationships, negotiation and compromise are not always easy. Expectations are not always met. The maintenance of a successful partnership requires ongoing negotiation and reflection. Critical analysis is an integral part of this negotiation. The establishment of the profession of midwifery in New Zealand also has been fraught with hostility from the medical profession and lack of understanding by some management structures that birth is a normal, healthy life event and that midwives are competent and capable of attending women on their own responsibility. Many midwives, too, have felt displaced and undervalued because they are unable to make the transition to independent practice. Mentor relationships have become essential within midwifery at every level as midwives support each other and work toward caseloads rather than "duties."

Since 1990, midwives in New Zealand have achieved radical change by collectively and enthusiastically acting on women's expressed need to demedicalize their birth experiences. They have only been able to achieve this because of the mentoring relationship between and among women and midwives. They will maintain this newfound professionalism only if they keep faith with women and provide the services they need and want. The foundation for success is the personal and professional partnerships between midwife and client. We believe success is the increased confidence, joy, and self-esteem that control over one's life brings. Empowerment sustains women in claiming their rightful place in society. Empowerment that comes through mentoring allows women to realize their potential for self-determination. The mentoring partnership enjoyed by women and midwives has played an essential role in the evolution and empowerment of New Zealand women and their maternity services.

The Philippine Nurses' Network

by Marie F. Santiago

MENTORING: A GOAL OF THE PHILIPPINE NURSES' NETWORK

For several years, I had a vision of creating an organization designed specifically for Filipino nurses whose members could enjoy collegial relationships by mentoring, inspiring, supporting and empowering each other. My vision was sparked at the height of the nursing shortage in the late 1980s, when large numbers of nurses were recruited from foreign countries to work in understaffed hospitals and nursing homes. Teaching students in the clinical setting enabled me to see the frustrations experienced by newly arrived nurses from the Philippines and other countries. They were working in a strange and new workplace, carrying heavy patient assignments, while at the same time going through the acculturation process and dealing with homesickness. I invited these nurses to attend a meeting for the purpose of networking and discussing their concerns. The first meeting in the

Fall of 1991 planted the seeds for what would eventually be called the Philippine Nurses' Network (PNN). Together with two Filipino nurse colleagues who, like me, have resided and worked in the United States for more than 20 years, the new immigrant nurses shared their feelings and concerns with us. They perceived a need to have a support group of experienced Filipino nurses who would mentor them. PNN would thus serve mentoring and networking functions. I took a leadership role in organizing the group and became PNN's founding president. During the first 6 months of PNN's founding, we recruited new members, established an organizational structure, formulated goals and bylaws, established working committees, began a newsletter, *The Network Chronicle*, and scheduled an inaugural dinner dance for induction of the officers. We envisioned a regional organization that would serve as a forum for mentoring, networking, resource sharing, advocacy, and professional development. An advisory board provided advice and assisted in mentoring members. I quickly became a mentor for a group of 12 officers who met with me on a monthly basis.

Mentoring Filipino nurses has been a truly enriching and empowering experience. Being a Filipino-American nurse with many years of education and experience in the United States has helped me be an effective mentor. The mentoring and professional development processes tapped into the unique resources and qualifications of each officer. In its 6 years of existence, PNN has succeeded in providing its members with mentoring opportunities; leadership and organizational skill development; access to a variety of educational, sociocultural, and professional activities; resource sharing, support, and recognition; and a chance to work with a dynamic, creative, and committed team. As an ethnic organization, it fosters and enhances cultural diversity within the nursing profession.

Lilibeth, a 26-year-old Filipino nurse, began working on a medical-surgical unit in a community hospital immediately after her arrival from the Philippines. Feeling lonely and homesick, Lilibeth sought the company and friendship of the other Filipinos who lived in the same residence hall. But, to her amazement, these nurses were all too busy working overtime to send money to support their families back home. One day, an acquaintance invited Lilibeth to attend a meeting of the PNN. Lilibeth subsequently became one of eight founding members of the network.

She became actively involved in helping to build the organization and agreed to serve as the first treasurer. The network's founder/president eventually became her mentor.

Lilibeth's case is a common situation for many newly arrived, foreign-born nurses who find themselves working in a strange land, without friends and support systems who can facilitate their acculturation to the host culture. Fortunately, Lilibeth's new friend, who was also an immigrant nurse, introduced her to other nurses who belonged to the new PNN. Soon Lilibeth found herself enjoying network activities, such as attending meetings, planning educational conferences and social functions, and formulating bylaws. As Lilibeth's mentor, I found myself in several roles: *adviser, communicator,* and *advocate.* Lilibeth and I worked on the formulation of her career goals for the next 5 years. Her plan was to work as a staff nurse for 4 years and then explore entry into graduate school, which would prepare her for an advanced practice nursing role. She also dreamed of the possibility of marriage and starting a family in combination with her career. In the *adviser* role, I recommended opportunities for Lilibeth's career training—she would need to obtain clinical experience in perioperative nursing, especially if she pursued the nurse anesthetist track. We discussed career options, such as obtaining a transfer to the operating room, or working in an ambulatory surgery unit of the postanesthesia care unit. We identified career obstacles and how to take appropriate actions to overcome these. The *communicator* role of my mentorship was challenging because of Lilibeth's personality: she was shy, soft-spoken, and demure. I consistently encouraged two-way exchanges of information between us. We established an atmosphere in which she could express her thoughts. I called her by telephone once a week so that we could maintain regular communication. Although it took Lilibeth some time to verbalize her concerns, she eventually responded positively to all my efforts. I used this experience to teach her about effective communication strategies, which she found valuable. Being an *advocate* for Lilibeth entailed taking an active interest on her behalf, offering her consistent praise and encouragement. She would relate work-related issues that bothered her.

There were times when we would disagree about modes of action, but we always discussed problem solving and conflict resolution strategies that she could use in a professional, ethical, and assertive manner. I also arranged for my protégé to participate in highly visible activities within the organization and outside of it. In monthly network officers' meetings, Lilibeth was placed on the agenda to give the treasurer's report. Whenever there are social functions, such as fund-raising events, I make sure that Lilibeth is seen center stage as mistress of ceremonies. Being treasurer of the network also places her in a high official position within the organization. Every task or function that was delegated to Lilibeth was an intervention for building self-esteem and confidence and to aid her personal and professional development.

POSTSCRIPT

I continue to serve as Lilibeth's mentor and to others in the network. It is my hope to continue to influence them as they embark on their respective journeys toward career specialization and professional advancement. My own professional life has been enriched by this mentorship. My protégés tell me that I serve as an inspiration and a role model to them. Lilibeth has asked me to share with her the "recipe" for success in combining marriage, motherhood, and an academic career. My experiences as both a mentor and protégé have made me realize the enormous value of the mentor relationship for both roles. When I reflect on my own experiences as a novice educator, I remember with special fondness and gratitude the encouragement that my own mentor provided. She was a nurse educator who provided me with numerous challenges in designing and teaching continuing education courses and allowed me to take risks. Without her guidance, I would not have been able to develop the teaching skills that paved my way toward a deeply satisfying career. Establishing mentor relationships has proven to be beneficial for my protégés and for me as mentor. Helping novice colleagues reach their career goals by mentoring them has increased my own self-confidence and leadership abilities. Furthermore, the mentor role provides the intellectual and scholarly stimulation that contributes continually to my career satisfaction. For my protégés, the inspiration provided by the mentor facilitates professional growth and a willingness to take risks. The nurturing relationship between mentor and protégé enhances the protégé's emotional support, increases self-confidence, and opens up new worlds of opportunities. Mentoring is a mutually empowering phenomenon.

Mentoring Experiences at the Academy for Nursing Studies in India

by M. Prakasamma

THE SITUATION

The Academy for Nursing Studies is a voluntary organization of nurses committed to improving the quality of nursing in India. The academy consists of clinical nurses, nurse educators, administrators, and practitioners who came together with the common aim of enhancing nursing education and practice through collaboration and coordination with the government, nursing associations, and other organizations in India and abroad. This is the first organization of this kind in India. Two newsletters have been distributed to 10,000 auxiliary nurse-midwives in the state, and we have prepared modules and supervisory formats for use by the health supervisors. The strategies we have adopted for achieving our goals are: (a) conducting continuing education; (b) developing standards; (c) preparing training modules and materials; and (d) providing guidelines to health and hospital administrators (governmental and private) on standards of nursing education and service. At the same time, we are reaching out to nurses to sensitize them to quality care and to reawaken the core of professional nursing in them. Seminars, conferences, newsletters, and small group interactions are very effective in reaching out to nurses. Their response has been gratifying. We have been approached by the Andhra Pradesh Vaidya Vidhana Parishad (APVVP)—a secondary-level medical department in the state government that employs about 4,000 nurses—to design an in-service training for staff nurses in their hospitals spread across India. We will conduct a training-needs assessment, design the training program, prepare training modules in 10 clinical areas, and train the core trainers.

THE PROCESS

We adopted the mentoring process for the entire program. The APVVP was requested to identify trainers and to place them with the Academy for Nursing Studies so that they would work along with us and learn the practical skills in designing and conducting a training program. Six nurses with B.Sc. and M.Sc. nursing qualifications were identified by the APVVP and sent to our organization. They would organize and conduct in-service training for nurses in the state, train other trainers for different regions within the state, and provide consultancy and guidance services. Mentoring would facilitate this work. The consultants at the academy are a small group of three dedicated nurses; one is a clinical practitioner, another is an educator, and the third is a researcher. All three are respected in the field of nursing for their involvement and dedication. The six trainers were welcomed to the organization and introduced to the mentoring partnership.

MENTORSHIP IN THE INDIAN CONTEXT

Mentorship is closely associated with the ancient Indian system of education. The *Guru-Shishya* relationship is considered the ideal mentor-student relationship. The teacher is usually a highly placed master in his or her field, committed to a cause. The student considers it a privilege to be accepted as a student. Each teacher takes only a few students who live close to the teacher, and observe, participate, and assist in his or her daily activities. The student learns not only from what the teacher says, but also from observing how the teacher behaves. The association between the two is a lasting personal relationship. The student displays loyalty to the teachings of the teacher and spreads the message further, and the teacher remains obligated to help the student. We found mentoring to be very effective in the qualitative training of the six nurses. Since they were to be leaders and trainers for the entire state, we felt that they should possess qualities that cannot be developed through formal classroom teaching. Working closely with someone whose sincerity and involvement are highly respected was considered essential to the development of the students' value systems. Though we had used mentoring previously with nurses and women organizers, we had done so as individuals. This was our first attempt at systematically adopting the process in an organization. The trainers initially stayed with us for 4 months. Close interaction occurred between the consultants and the trainers. We discussed late into the evening; most sessions were informal; planning was done together; and personal experiences in nursing were shared. They observed our consultants at work and how they interacted with each other for a common goal.

OBSERVED OUTCOMES

During the last month of the protégé-trainers' stay with us, we could see a visible change in their outlook. Though the six trainers had initially come to the APVVP with various personal motives, their perception of the program had slowly undergone a change. The mentors were beginning to be treated not just as teachers to be respected, but as friendly seniors who could be approached for guidance later. The changes include:

Pride in the profession.

Working with experienced and qualified nurses who deal with nursing issues with confidence and concern helps the protégés feel more comfortable as nurses. In India, nursing is not considered the first choice as a career, and the image of nursing is low. We in the Academy for Nursing Studies believe that the first change required for improving nursing is an acceptance of and pride in the profession.

Sensitivity and concern.

Experience sharing is one of the major processes being used to train nurse leaders. The clinical nurse specialist on the team relates her experiences with patients and relatives, role plays are conducted, and the trainers are encouraged to respond. Nurses' behavior with patients and others is openly discussed and analyzed.

Leadership development.

Negotiation activities and collaboration with different organizations were arranged so that the protégés could see how their mentors talk with nursing and health administrators. Each of them learned to work independently under the mentor's guidance.

Systematic organization and management.

The protégé-trainers conducted a 1-day seminar for head nurses and nursing superintendents on "Nursing Supervision for Quality Patient Care." They planned the requirements for the in-service training center after their training with us.

Trainer development.

We could see a big difference in the methodology and approach to training in the six candidates. They were encouraged to observe closely the sessions conducted by the mentors and to comment on them and evaluate them. They learned to use different methods for achieving different objectives.

OUR EXPECTATIONS

- We trust that our protégés will be self-confident and capable of planning and conducting in-service training for the nearly 4,000 staff nurses for whom they are being prepared. We hope they will become leaders in nursing since they will be at the training apex in India.
- We are preparing our protégés to view nursing as a human relations profession within a science-based practice. We hope that they will use these principles and thus direct nursing in the state toward a more humane process.
- We expect our protégés to be our links with clinical nurses and become their mentors in promoting awareness and interest for professional nursing behavior. Our message of nursing values will be spread through these mentor-leaders.
- We will use our protégés as resource persons when the Academy for Nursing Studies conducts programs for in-service education, preparation of modules, and textbooks, setting standards, and conducting conferences. We hope that the strong mentor relationships built between us will continue to motivate them to participate in all our activities.
- We hope to get feedback from our protégés on clinical situations and to interact with the nurses from small-town and district hospitals through these leaders. This will provide clinical material for our own growth.

FUTURE PLANS

- We will be conducting regular "mentoring interactions" in the future and hope to have five students always with us to develop into nursing leaders, to train as trainers, to develop as mentors, counselors,

and human relations resource persons. We are collabo-
rating with other institutes in this regard.
- We plan to launch a journal for clinical nurses in simple language about the various aspects of nursing. At
the present, there is only one professional journal for
nurses in India.
- We are planning to write books for nurses in the Indian
context. At the present, most of our textbooks are from
the United States or Great Britain. Although they are
excellent in content, the practical examples and cases are
not clearly understood or culturally relevant.
- We plan to begin a few action-oriented projects in
nursing to show improvements in the clinical and
community situations. Projects on home care nursing
and rehabilitation are being reviewed.

CONCLUSION

We believe that the mentor process has been effective in goal
achievement in a short time. This has been a golden opportunity
for us to make a dent in the apathy and lethargy in nursing in the
state. Our aims were to mold these six nurses—our protégés—into
change agents for nursing in the state of Andhra Pradesh. A lot
was at stake for us. We were testing our own value systems and
concerns for nursing. How we mentored these protégés would
eventually influence how they would mentor trainee staff nurses.
We found the process of mentoring personally rewarding since it
helped further the growth of our inner selves. It was professionally
satisfying since it sharpened our skills and gave us a means
through which we could reach other nurses. It established nursing
networks in every part of the state. Mentoring helped us to achieve
a striking shift in the attitudes and value systems of our six nurse-
protégés that will further influence nurses throughout India.

**A Study of Mentoring and Career Development of Directors of
Nursing in South Australia**

by Grant Sharples

The mentor experiences in the career development of directors of
nursing in South Australia were surveyed in relation to fre-

quency, qualities, and dimensions of mentor relationships. Questionnaires were sent to a random sample of 100 directors of nursing in South Australia with a response rate of 77%. The majority (83%) of directors of nursing were female with a mean age of 45 years. More than half the participants (60%) reported having a mentor at some point in their professional lives, either as undergraduates, postgraduates (when undertaking specialty training), or later as managers. Consistent with reports of mentoring in the business world, mentoring was most prevalent in the early years of professional development. Most subjects did not have a mentor while serving as a director of nursing, reporting that they had gone beyond the stage when a mentor was valuable and that they were "self-contained." These senior nurses used networking as a means of career development, making use of their expanded range of contacts. Directors of nursing with no experience as mentors said that "mentoring was not a popular concept at the time of my training (25 years ago)" and "they did not need a mentor." One director said, "As an intelligent human being, I learned from those I was in contact with, adopting skills and knowledge from a large number of people . . . selecting the good points I liked." The evolving career focus of the protégé was reflected in the professional position held by the mentor.

Initially, mentors were found from the midcareer professionals in nursing, including charge nurses, nurse supervisors, and educators. Later, nurses received the support of other directors of nursing and from mentors outside the discipline, usually male chief executive officers. The nature of these relationships was essentially the same throughout the nurse's career development. These mentor-protégé relationships were voluntary rather than arranged by an employer. Respondents reported that the relationships were mutually initiated, with the inexperienced person seeking help and the senior professional offering assistance. Feelings of trust and respect emerged. Mentors contributed to the nursing directors' job satisfaction, knowledge, skills, and career progress. Mentors were usually held in high regard. The most frequently reported valued traits of mentors were competence and intelligence. Other characteristics ascribed to the mentors were friendliness, honesty, sensitivity, credibility, compassion, and nonjudgmental attitude.

True to the spirit of mentoring, the relationships described by subjects ($N = 77$)were long lived, typically spanning at least 5 years. Protégés reported that most mentor relationships (79%) ended on pleasant terms, with the protégé and mentor drifting apart as a result of relocation, transfer, or retirement. Indeed, the majority of participants indicated that they had remained in contact with their mentors, who are now regarded as friends. This result differs from the Levinson, Darrow, Klein, Levinson, and McKee (1978) study in which male mentors and protégés "formed, normed and stormed." This contradiction may be due to gender differences or reflection of a nurturing nature among nurses. What transpired when a mentor relationship ended? Some nurses pursued another mentor and had several mentors throughout their career history. Similarly, former protégés reported supporting the professional development of less experienced coworkers. There is a widespread mentoring ethic among directors of nursing, with many (70%) actively assisting junior nurses. They state that "mentoring is part of my professional role"; it "fosters teamwork"; and "contributes to a well-run hospital." There also is evidence of a strong, mentoring generational legacy among directors of nursing. Those who had a mentor were more likely to support the career of others than nonmentored nurses. The stimulus to mentor others may be a response to the kindness shown protégés during their careers. It is important to note that being a mentor is intrinsically rewarding. The mentor gains personal satisfaction from the relationship. The act of nurturing becomes a source of pride, accomplishment, and positive feedback. Mentors derive "satisfaction" and "renewed enthusiasm" from the experience. In the words of some directors of nursing, "it was nice to pass it on"; "I enjoyed sharing my skills . . . helping others pursue their career and success." One director described mentoring as "uplifting . . . almost spiritual." Directors of nursing who were not actively assisting others often felt constrained by the pressures of office. Some nurses believed that mentoring may be seen as favoritism by others. Many wrote that they have "heavy workloads" and that "there is no time to mentor others." One person stated that, in her experience, "the health system is demanding it, but doesn't acknowledge the time and commitment given to mentoring."

CONCLUSION

This study provides evidence of a mentoring legacy among nurses in Australia. This legacy is founded, in part, on the benefits that mentoring has for both the mentor and protégé and to the nursing profession and organizations. Mentoring also is congruent with a caring profession, embodying as it does mutual trust, support, and respect. Ironically, at a time when economic constraints may be a threat to mentoring by senior nurses, there is an enormous need for nurses to support and mentor one another.

Mentorship in Italy

by Renzo Zanotti

HISTORIC OVERVIEW

Nursing education in Italy has a tradition that goes back to the first professional nursing school established in 1920. Mentorship was formally defined as a professional activity in 1975, according to a European agreement dictating the requirements for nursing education. The mentor, as defined by the agreement, was a nurse with high-level clinical expertise who was in charge of the student protégé's clinical training and who functioned as a link with the academic setting. To be an effective link, the nurse-mentors had to be assigned as faculty to the school. As a consequence, nursing schools had to recruit clinical nurses, mainly from hospital wards, to serve as mentors to support students' training and education. Two concepts emerged about the mentor's educational role:

1. The mentor was viewed as connected to the group of students; therefore, the mentor followed the group wherever it went. The mentor's clinical expertise was considered less important than educational skills. The mentor had to be a creator of learning opportunities for the students.
2. The mentor was viewed as a true nurse specialist, a "master" in his or her area of activity and therefore tied to a specific clinical setting. The mentor's educational skills were important, but clinical expertise was paramount. The mentor was a clinical model, a reference point within the training hospital wards.

Those two concepts received almost equal support among the mentors, and for many years created criticism and debate. However, in the long run, the second viewpoint was most prevalent. The late 1970s were a period of unrecognized mentors' heroic commitment. The first mentors, generally staff and head nurses, without any recognition as teachers, developed programs and textbooks, in the absence of official literature. Moreover, often without a background in education, they had to choose appropriate teaching methods in class and in clinical settings, define common educational goals, and coordinate other teachers to achieve the established objectives. They all put enthusiasm and dedication in the job. Little by little the mentors achieved an acceptable status within the health services system. However, the role became more connected with academic teaching, almost synonymous with "nurse teacher."

ARE ITALIAN NURSES ATTRACTED BY MENTORSHIP?

A mentor in Italy has less income and more duties to accomplish than a clinical staff nurse. Why are nurses attracted to this role? There are some personally gratifying aspects. Being a mentor places a person in the spotlight by students and colleagues, thus increasing self-esteem and respect. Mentoring offers many stimuli by providing a variety of teaching and learning opportunities, and cultural relationships. However, there are challenges: additional responsibilities, unexpected activities, high student expectations, and an unclear role. These reasons explain why mentorship is difficult in Italy. Mentorship may mean less power, detachment from the clinical setting, and a temporary engagement. What is most attractive is the possibility to be connected with academia, to fulfill basic requirements for a future professorship, or to influence future nurses.

In 1992, nursing education started to move toward the university system. Although nursing is considered a separate discipline, it was incorporated into the School of Medicine, a process that was completed in 1996, when the hospital nursing schools were closed. Mentors will play a key role in the new educational system. Because of the bureaucratic way in which Italian universities are managed, the need for leadership across clinical training settings requires strong mentorship. An even more important reason to predict the future value and need for mentorship is that it is the mentor who is a role model for students, an exemplar of how the student is expected to perform as a future professional and leader. In the Italian universities, nursing professors are considered by the students as a point of reference for the discipline culture, not for professional practice. Therefore, nursing students need to be coached in the clinical settings by nurse-mentors to apply what they have learned and to understand what it means "to be a nurse who cares for people."

CONCLUSION

Only a highly professional culture allows a nurse to be a good mentor for students; thus culture is a requisite as well as professional practice for mentorship. A mentor should lead students in experimenting, selecting options, and using alternative approaches in daily professional activities. A mentor should be a living expression of a trustworthy mix of culture and experience—a reliable guide among difficult decisions and uncertainty. Can a nurse be a good mentor without being prepared for mentorship? Perhaps, but only if she or he possesses highly professional preparation, experience gained under excellent teachers and mentors, and vision and commitment to professional practice. I prefer to think that mentorship is an ensemble of professional attitudes, personal experience, and values, and that this delicate and complex role requires unique sensitivity, knowledge, and skills.

A Russian-American Tale of Mentoring

by Irina Ivancovich, Nurse Midwife

Could it be possible for a Russian nurse to have a mentor from a different country—from an entirely different social system—from another world? I am a nurse from Russia, and my mentor is a nurse from the United States. For many years, America was closed to us Russians. It was in 1990 that I became acquainted with American health care, the educational system, and the professional level of American nurses. During the breakup of the Communist system, relations between our countries became more open and trusting, and a large wave of student and professional exchanges began. However, any idea about continuing my nursing education and developing a nursing career was still a dream. Instead, my thoughts centered on the dissatisfaction in my work, the low professional and social status of Russian nurses, and the absence of any possibilities for professional growth. In childhood, a girl's mentor is often her mother, who prepares her for a future independent life. My mother, observing my "hospital doll games" saw in me a future nurse. After graduation from a nursing school in Leningrad, I had a nurse-mentor who taught me professional skills and helped me work out various problems. However, professional growth was possible only in self-education, because the idea of a nursing career did not exist. I didn't have any sense of what it would mean to have a true professional mentor. However, subconsciously, I was looking for a mentor who would share with me life experiences, wisdom, and knowledge and try to prevent me from taking wrong steps. In the past, such a person would be known as a teacher. Now I understand and deeply value what it means to have a mentor. I first met my American mentor, Connie Vance, while she was visiting and consulting with Russian hospitals and nursing schools. I came to know her better when I participated in a professional exchange program for 4 months at her college in New York. I lived in her home with her children and became part of her family life. She came to be not only my mentor but a close friend. We two nurses from two very different countries found many similarities between us. My mentor shared with me her energy, love of life and of nursing, and gave me a new self-confidence. I saw the career-lifestyle of my mentor and other nurses who were teachers, midwives, and clinical nurses. I went to classes with my American peers and found their dreams, goals, and worries to be the same as mine. My mentor helped me trust my future and potential. I began to see myself more clearly, to find my own path, and to aspire to new goals. The most important thing I discovered was that it is possible to have dreams that someone else believes in and to be on the move toward them.

A few Faculties of Highest Nursing Education have been established recently in Russia, and I have become a student at one of them in St. Petersburg. Many plans and ideas call me forward, such as starting a birth center and a midwifery association. I decided to demonstrate how new ideas can work and to use myself as an example of how a midwife can practice in a new role. I have started a small model of a new perinatal service in clinics and a birth house. An American midwifery expert and colleague, Ruth Lubic, suggested that I begin with a women's health education project, where women can learn about the maintenance of healthy bodies, nutrition, exercise, the pregnancy and birth process, and infant and family care. My mentor is assisting me in the support of this project through the sale of hand-painted Russian brooches. With these funds, we have purchased a tape recorder, videocassettes, a television set, a pager, a birthing stool, books, and supplies. I currently follow a caseload of pregnant couples, providing them with support and classes, and assist in their deliveries. I also provide lectures at the midwifery college from where I graduated. Several of the students work with me as interns, take my classes, and refer women to my service. It is my dream to expand this model through the mentorship of nurse midwives, the formation of a birth center, and developing a strong professional association of nurse midwives. My American mentors and I are seeking funding to achieve these goals. American and Russian women face the same concerns about family, work and social life, health, economics, and the desire to better their lives. Our mutual sharing, mentorship, and partnering provide inspiration and courage for greater world understanding and help us take action to improve our lives and our professional work. I believe that the development of strong bonds among women and nurses across the world will occur through our mentor relationships. These bonds will help us raise the standard of health care and nursing education in all our countries.

Epilogue

In the final analysis, mentoring has everything to do with developing together, to think, to feel, to learn and to grow. It is ultimately to do with the human spirit and how we cherish that within ourselves and within others (McIntyre, Hagger & Wilkin, 1993).

As we "touch tomorrow" through the legacy of our mentor relationships (Kelly, 1987), we have a precious opportunity to take stock of where we are headed in our personal and professional growth journeys. It will become increasingly important to assess the changing environment and our relationship to it. Many believe that the "second curve"of the future will irrevocably alter the way every profession and organization will function (Morrison, 1996). We know, for example, that old-order (command-and-control hierarchical) organizations are being replaced by organizational web structures of networks, alliances, and mentor connections. These structures can respond rapidly and creatively to change and restructuring. Learning organizations are evolving that incorporate the precepts of mentoring into their everyday value systems, support structures, and working relationships. They are thus able to expand their ability to create their future by tapping people's capacity to learn at all levels in the organization. Meaning and commitment are strengthened.

Feminine principles are entering the public realm in response to a changing world. They are redefining education, family life, work, leadership, and mentorship. New forms of relationships, including mentoring, partnering, and networking, are becoming essential for development and mastery through the career-life journey in an evolving environment. The mentor connection provides us with unsurpassed, and frequently unimagined, opportunities for nurturing the growth of our colleagues and students. Each of us will be a beneficiary. Our mentor connections will foster both our individual and collective power. They will provide us with new meaning and purpose. Mentoring assists us in the creation of new models for achieving and sharing, for reconstructing value systems, and humanizing organizations and professions. Building mentor connections is a transformational act. These connections should not be an isolated phenomenon and it should be integrated into one's daily professional life.

LESSONS FOR THE FUTURE

CREATE A CULTURE OF LEARNING AND MENTORING—IN THE WORKPLACE AND IN SCHOOLS

Active mentoring of colleagues and students is an investment in the future. The full success and satisfaction of professional persons relies heavily on the presence of learning cultures composed of caring colleagues. Both informal mentoring and formal mentor programs are ingredients of a learning culture. The survival and development of the professions and organizations, now in the midst of massive and fundamental change, will depend upon changing the patterns of interaction between people and processes. Developing peoples' capacities to think and interact differently will require active mentoring and learning among colleagues and students. Structural changes in educational and clinical environments must be created so that nurturing and caring can exist among nurses and their clients-patients.

BUILD A LEGACY OF MENTORING

The mentoring of a protégé creates a new mentor who will then pass on the heritage and gift of mentoring to others. This generational network will assist in the evolution of new relational structures in organizations and professional life. These structures will be built on a foundation of mutual respect, trust, encouragement, and empowerment. Since the empowerment and care of others are leadership tasks, evolving organizations (whether they be educational, clinical, or corporate) will require leaders who consciously foster the mentorship and development of others.

MENTOR AS PYGMALION

Act on the power of expectation with colleagues and students. Search faithfully for your own and others' gifts, and find avenues for polishing special talents. Mentors see potential, often unacknowledged by others. They have visions of a new future for a profession and its practitioners. Mentors can inspire and empower protégés to acknowledge their visions and dreams through periods of change and challenge.

GIVE VOICE TO MENTORING

Share stories with students, neophytes, peers, and leaders. Give voice to your own story. Stories provide encouragement and guideposts for others. "The joining of visions and voices creates something new, an enlarged vision. The sense of connection and participation . . . heightens the sense of personal power and understanding" (Surrey, 1991). Exploring new realities and new ways of "knowing" through sharing our voices will further strengthen our mentoring.

CREATE INNOVATIVE APPROACHES TO MENTORING

Act on an expanded conception of mentoring that includes a variety of learning partners. Establish a repertoire of different mentors for different seasons and for different reasons. The new paradigm of mentoring is androgynous, embodying both traditional and evolving patterns of helping and supporting. Be both mentor and protégé, understanding the necessity for continuous learning and growth for oneself and for others. Develop a mind-set of mentoring wherever you are—remembering that mentoring is an attitude of mind *and* heart. Seek opportunities to mentor: listening, encouraging, and sharing are gifts that inspire and energize.

SUMMARY

The construction of a new paradigm of mentor connections will require innovative pioneers. The status quo in formal and informal mentor relationships should be challenged through the creation of new ways of participating in the development of each other and sharing our gifts of heart and mind. Through these personal and professional partnerships, the unique differences and contributions of each individual, regardless of gender, age, ethnicity, culture, and race, will be acknowledged and celebrated. It is our belief that through the simple, yet powerful, human phenomenon of mentorship, even one caring, involved, interested person can make a difference in another person's life. This difference will be reflected ultimately in professional practice, in the care and education of our students and patients, and in organizational life and the value systems of society.

References and Bibliography

Aburdene, P., & Naisbitt, J. (1992). *Megatrends for women.* New York: Villard Books.

Aisenberg, N., & Harrington, M. (1988). *Women of academe: Outsiders in the sacred grove.* Amherst, MA: University of Massachusetts Press.

Altieri, L. B., & Elgin, P. A. (1994). A decade of nursing leadership research. *Holistic Nurse Practice, 9*(1), 75–82.

Alvarez, A., & Abriam-Yago, K. (1993). Mentoring undergraduate ethnic-minority students: A strategy for retention. *Journal of Nursing Education, 32*(5), 230–232.

Andrica, D. C. (1996). Mentoring: Executive responsibility? *Nursing Economics, 14*(2), 128.

Angelini, D. J. (1995). Mentoring in the career development of hospital staff nurses: Models and strategies. *Journal of Professional Nursing, 11*(2) 89–97.

Ardery, G. (1990). Mentors and protégés: From idealogy to knowledge. In J. McCloskey & H. Grace (Eds.), *Current issues in nursing* (pp. 58–63). St. Louis: Mosby.

Arnoldussen, B., & White, L. M. (1990). The mentoring experience. *Nursing Administration Quarterly, 15*(1), 28–35.

Astin, H. S., & Leland, C. (1991). *Women of influence, women of vision: A cross-generational study of leaders and social change.* San Francisco: Jossey-Bass.

Atkins, S., & Williams, A. (1995). Registered nurses' experiences of mentoring undergraduate nursing students. *Journal of Advanced Nursing, 21,*1006–1015.

Atwood, A. H. (1979). The mentor in clinical practice. *Nursing Outlook, 27,* 714–717.

Atwood, A. H. (1981). Effects of a three-month mentorship on mentors and new graduate nurses in an acute-care urban hospital (Doctoral dissertation, University of San Francisco, 1981). *Dissertation Abstracts International, 42,* 3817A.

Atwood, A. H. (1986). *Mentoring: A paradigm for nursing.* Los Altos, CA: National Nursing Review.

Bahr, J. E. (1985). Mentoring experiences of women administrators in baccalaureate nursing education (Doctoral dissertation, Oklahoma State University, 1985). *Dissertation Abstracts International, 47,* 798A.

Bahti, M. (1988). *Pueblo stories and storytellers.* Tucson, AZ: Treasure Chest Publications, Inc.

Baker, C., & Diekelmann, N. (1994). Connecting conversations of caring: Recalling the narrative to clinical practice. *Nursing Outlook, 42,* 65–70.

Baldwin, D., & Wold, J. (1993a, April). Matching mentors and protégés in nursing education: Strategies that work. *Proceedings from the Diversity in Mentoring Conference,* Atlanta, GA: 25–39.

Baldwin, D., & Wold, J. (1993b). Students from disadvantaged backgrounds: Satisfaction with a mentor-protégé relationship. *Journal of Nursing Education, 32*(5), 225–226.

Bamford, P., Hullstrung, R., & Niedzwiecki, G. (1997). Developing caring connections: nursing Students, alumni, and faculty. In International Mentoring Association. *Diversity in Mentoring,* (pp. 134–140). Kalamazoo, MI: Western Michigan University.

Bandura, A. (1977). *Social learning theory.* Englewood Cliffs, NJ: Prentice-Hall.

Barnshaw, G. J. (1995). Mentorship: The students' views. *Nurse Education Today, 15*(4), 274–279.

Bateson, M. C. (1990). *Composing a life.* New York: Penguin.

Beaulieu, L. P. (1988). Preceptorship and mentorship: Bridging the gap between nursing education and nursing practice. *Imprint, 35*(2), 111, 113, 115.

Becker, H., & Strauss, A. (1956). Careers, personality, and adult socialization. *American Journal of Sociology, 62,* 253–265.

Belenky, M. F., Clinchy, B. M., Goldberger, N. R., & Tarule, J. M. (1986). *Women's ways of knowing: The development of self, voice, and mind.* New York: Basic Books.

Benner, P. (1984). *From novice to expert: Excellence and power in clinical nursing practice.* Menlo Park, CA: Addison-Wesley.

Benner, P. (1991). The role of experience, narrative, and community in skilled ethical comportment. *Advances in Nursing Science, 14*(2), 1–21.

Bessent, H. (1989). Postdoctoral leadership training for women of color. *Journal of Professional Nursing, 5,* 279–282.

Bidwell, A. S., & Brasler, M. L. (1989). Role modeling versus mentoring in nursing education. *Image: Journal of Nursing Scholarship, 21*(1), 23–25.

Bolen, J. S. (1985). *Goddesses in every woman: A new psychology of women.* New York: Harper & Row.

Bolton, E. B. (1980). A conceptual analysis of the mentoring relationship in the career development of women. *Adult Education, 30*(4), 195–207.

Borman, J. S. (1993). Women and nurse executives: Finally, some advantages.

Journal of Nursing Administration, 23(10), 34–41.

Boyer, E. L. (1990). *Scholarship reconsidered: Priorities of the professoriate.* Lawrenceville, NJ: Carnegie Foundation for the Advancement of Teaching.

Boykin, A., & Schoenhofer, S. O. (1991). Story as link between nursing practice, ontology, epistemology. *Image: Journal of Nursing Scholarship, 23*(4), 245–248.

Boykin, A., & Schoenhofer, S. (1993). *Nursing as caring: A model for transforming practice.* New York: National League for Nursing.

Boyle, C., & James, S. K. (1990). Nursing leaders as mentors: How are we doing? *Nursing Administration Quarterly, 15*(1), 44–48.

Brito, H. H. (1992). Nurses in action: An innovative approach to mentoring. *Journal of Nursing Administration, 22*(5), 22–28.

Brykczynski, K. A. (1993). Response to "nurse practitioner-patient discourse: Uncovering the voice of nursing in primary care practice." *Scholarly Inquiry for Nursing Practice: An International Journal, 7*(3), 159–163.

Buchanan, J. (1993). The student-teacher relationship: The heart of nursing education. In N. Dieckelman & M. Ratner (Eds.), *Transforming nursing R.N. education: Dialogue and debate.* National League for Nursing, Publication No. 14–2511, 304–323.

Bucher, R., & Steeling, J. G. (1977). *Becoming professional.* Beverly Hills, CA: Sage.

Budhos, M. (1996). Mentoring women graduate students. *Monthly Forum on Women in Higher Education, 1*(4), 13–14.

Burnard, P. (1990). The student experience: Adult learning and mentorship revisited. *Nurse Education Today, 10,* 349–354.

Burns, J. M. (1978). *Leadership.* New York: Harper & Row.

Butler, M. J. (1989). Mentoring and scholarly productivity in nursing faculty (Doctoral dissertation, West Virginia University, 1989). *Dissertation Abstracts International, 51,* 691.

Byrne, M. M., Kangas, S. K., & Warren, N. (1996). Advice for beginning nurse researchers. *Image: Journal of Nursing Scholarship, 28*(2), 165–167.

Cahill, M. F., & Kelly, J. J. (1989). A mentor program for nursing majors. *Journal of Nursing Education, 28*(1), 40–44.

Caine, R. M. (1989a). A comparative survey of mentoring and job satisfaction: Perceptions of clinical nurse specialists (Doctoral dissertation, Pepperdine University, 1989). *Dissertation Abstracts International, 50,* 1148A.

Caine, R. M. (1989b). Mentoring the novice clinical nurse specialist. *Clinical Nurse Specialist, 3*(2), 76–78.

Cameron, R. K. (1982). Wanted: Mentor relationships within nursing administration. *Nursing Leadership, 5*(1), 18–22.

Campbell, J. (1988). *The power of myth.* New York: Doubleday.

Campbell-Heider, N. (1986). Do nurses need mentors? *Image: Journal of*

Nursing Scholarship, 18(3), 110–113.

Carey, S. J., & Campbell, S. T. (1994). Preceptor, mentor, and sponsor roles: Creative strategies for nurse retention. *Journal of Nursing Administration, 24*(12), 39–48.

Carmin, C. N. (1988). Issues in research on mentoring: Definitional and methodological. *International Journal of Mentoring, 2*(2), 9–13.

Carrolton, E. T. (1989). Factors influencing career success of nursing leaders in hospitals (Doctoral dissertation, University of Connecticut, 1989). *Dissertation Abstracts International, 50,* 5544B.

Castiglia, P. (1996). Multidisciplinary care and education. In R. W. Richards (Ed.), *Building partnerships: Educating health professionals for the communities they serve* (pp. 157–171). San Francisco: Jossey-Bass.

Chamings, P. A., & Brown, B. J. (1984). The dean as mentor. *Nursing & Health Care, 5*(2), 88–91.

Clark, R. A. (1994). Mentoring relationships of men into academic role in nursing programs (Doctoral dissertation, University of Alabama at Birmingham, 1994). *Dissertation Abstracts International, 56,* 739B.

Clauson, J. B. (1980). Mentoring in managerial careers. In C. B. Derr (Ed.), *Work, family and the career* (pp. 144–165). New York: Praeger.

Clayton, G. M., Broome, M. E., & Ellis, L. A. (1989). Relationship between a preceptorship experience and role socialization of graduate nurses. *Journal of Nursing Education, 28*(2), 72–75.

Cockram, D. H. (1992). Profiles, functions, and career experiences of selected hospital nurse executives in the United States (Doctoral dissertation, Virginia Polytechnic Institute and State University, 1992). *Dissertation Abstracts International, 53,* 3416A.

Collins, B. A. (1993). A review and integration of knowledge about faculty research productivity. *Journal of Professional Nursing, 9*(3), 159–168.

Collins, E., & Scott, P. (1978). Everyone who makes it has a mentor. *Harvard Business Review, 56*(4), 89–101.

Collins, N. W. (1983). *Professional women and their mentors.* Englewood Cliffs, NJ: Prentice-Hall.

Conway, M. E., & Glass, L. K. (1978). Socialization for survival in the academic world. *Nursing Outlook, 26,* 424–429.

Cooper, M. D. (1990). Mentorship: The key to the future of professionalism in nursing. *Journal of Perinatal Neonatal Nursing, 4*(3), 71–77.

Cotton, P. (1992). Women scientists explore more ways to smash through the glass ceiling. *Journal of American Medical Association, 268*(2), 173.

Cullen, D. L., Rodak, B., Fitzgerald, N., & Baker, S. (1993). Minority students benefit from mentoring programs. *Radiologic Technology, 64*(4), 226–231.

Daloz, L. A. (1986). *Effective teaching and mentoring: Realizing the transformational power of adult learning experiences.* San Francisco: Jossey-Bass.

Dalton, G., Thompson, P., & Price, R. (1977, Summer). The four stages of professional careers. *Organizational Dynamics, 6,* 19–42.

Daly, J. M., & Jones, T. (1988). An independent study in conjunction with a sophomore nursing course. *Journal of Nursing Education, 27*(5), 231–232.

Darling, L. W. (1984). The mentoring dimension: What do nurses want in a mentor? *Journal of Nursing Administration, 14*(10), 42–44.

Davidhizar, R. E. (1988). Mentoring in doctoral education. *Journal of Advanced Nursing, 13,* 775–781.

dela Cruz, F. A., Jacobs, A. M., Villegas, L. M., & Mucci, P. A. (1994). *Final report of the high risk home health nursing clinical specialty program.* Azusa, CA: Azusa Pacific University School of Nursing.

DeMarco, R. (1993). Mentorship: A feminist critique of current research. *Journal of Advanced Nursing, 18,* 1242–1250.

Department of Health. (1990). *Nurses Amendment Act 1990. Information for health providers.* Wellington, New Zealand: Department of Health.

Dimino, E. (1986). *Senior BSN preceptorship in perioperative nursing.* Unpublished post-master's study, Old Dominion University, Norfolk, VA.

Dolan, J. A., Fitzpatrick, M. L., & Herrman, E. K. (1983). *Nursing in society: A historical perspective* (15th ed.). Philadelphia: Saunders.

Donley, J. (1986). *Save the midwife.* Auckland, New Zealand: New Women's Press.

Drucker, P. F. (1988). The coming of the new organization. *Harvard Business Review, 66*(1), 45–53.

Drucker, P. F. (1995). *Managing in a time of great change.* New York: Talley/ Dutton.

Duane, S. J. (1986). *Mentor-protégé relationships: A study of career development among graduate nursing students.* Unpublished master's thesis, State University of New York, Buffalo.

Duff, C. S., & Cohen, B. (1993). *When women work together: Using our strengths to overcome our challenges.* Berkeley, CA: Conari Press.

Dunsmore, J. M. (1987). *A study to examine the differences in job satisfaction and role clarity of unit managers in hospital settings who have had mentor relationships and those who have not.* Unpublished master's thesis, University of Washington, Seattle.

Epstein, C. F. (1970). *Women's place: Options and limits in professional careers.* Berkeley, CA: University of California Press.

Erikson, E. (1963). *Childhood and society* (3rd ed.). New York: Norton.

Erikson, E. (1968). *Identity: Youth and crisis.* New York: Norton.

Estes, C. P. (1992). *Women who run with the wolves: Myths and stories of the wild women archetype.* New York: Ballantine Books.

Fagan, M. M. (1988). The term mentor: A review of the literature and a pragmatic suggestion. *International Journal of Mentoring, 2*(2), 5–8.

Fagan, M., & Fagan, P. (1983). Mentoring among nurses. *Nursing & Health Care, 4*(2), 77–82.

Felton, G. (1978). On women, networks, patronage and sponsorship. *Image: Journal of Nursing Scholarship, 10*(3), 58–59.

Fenske, M. M. (1986). A comparison of the perceptions of mentoring relationships in the careers of female chief academic officers of nursing and male chief academic officers of education (Doctoral dissertation, Vanderbilt University, George Peabody College, 1986). *Dissertation Abstracts International, 47,* 2392A.

Fields, W. L. (1988). Analysis of the concept mentor. *International Journal of Mentoring, 2*(2), 14–19.

Fields, W. L. (1991). Mentoring in nursing: A historical approach. *Nursing Outlook, 39*(6), 257–261.

Fitzpatrick, J. J., & Abraham, I. L. (1987). Toward the socialization of scholars and scientists. *Nurse Educator, 12*(3), 172–176.

Fitzpatrick, M. L. (1991). Doctoral preparation versus expectations. *Journal of Professional Nursing, 7*(3), 172–176.

Fox, J. (1991). Mentorship and the charge nurse. *Nursing Standard, 5*(23), 34–36.

Freeman, S. (1989). The mentor experience as perceived by nurse practitioners: Implications for curriculum design (Doctoral dissertation, Georgia State University, 1989). *Dissertation Abstracts International, 51,* 67A.

Galbraith, L. K., Brueggemeyer, A. E., & Manweiler, D. L. (1988). Failure to flourish: Indications for mentoring. *Pediatric Nursing, 14*(5), 405–408.

Garner, E. E. (1995). Survival of the fittest: An ethnographic study of nurse administrators (Doctoral dissertation, Texas Woman's University, 1995). *Dissertation Abstracts International, 55,* 4320.

Gehrke, N. (1988). Toward a definition of mentoring. *Theory into Practice, 27*(3), 190–194.

Gerdes, H., & Mallinckrodt, B. (1994). Emotional, social, and academic adjustment of college students: A longitudinal study of retention. *Journal of Counseling & Development, 72,* 281–288.

Giese, J. (1986). *A study to explore the differences in job satisfaction between leaders in hospital settings who have had mentor relationships and those who have not.* Unpublished master's thesis, University of Washington, Seattle.

Gilligan, C. (1993). *In a different voice: Psychological theory and women's development (Rev. ed.).* Cambridge, MA: Harvard University Press. (1st ed. published in 1982)

Gioiella, E. C. (1993). Meeting the demands for advanced practice nurses. *Journal of Professional Nursing, 9*(5), 254.

Glynn, P., Arndt, M., Beal, J., & Bennett, N. (1996). The interconnectedness of nurses' lives: Implications for nursing management. *Journal of Nursing Administration, 26*(5), 36–42.

Gonzalez, L. (1994). Faculty mentors for minority undergraduate students. *Journal of Cultural Diversity, 1*(4), 90–94.

Goodnough-Hanneman, S. K., Bines, A. S., & Sajtar, W. S. (1993). The indirect patient care effect of a unit-based clinical nurse specialist on preventable pulmonary complications. *American Journal of Critical Care, 2,* 331–338.

Gresley, R. S. (1986). *The effect of mentorships in improving self-concept and professional role development in senior-level baccalaureate nursing students.* Postdoctoral unpublished study, Southern Illinois University, Edwardsville.

Guido-DiBrito, F., Noteboom, P. A., Nathan, L., & Fenty, J. (1996). Traditional and new paradigm leadership: The gender link. *Initiatives, 58*(1) 27–38.

Guilliland, K., & Pairman, S. (1995). *The midwifery partnership—A model for practice.* Wellington, New Zealand: Victoria University Monograph Series.

Haffer, A. G. (1990). Beginning nurses' diagnostic reasoning behaviors derived from observation and verbal protocol analysis (Doctoral dissertation, University of San Francisco, 1990). *Dissertation Abstracts International, 52,* 160B.

Hagerty, B. (1986). A second look at mentors. *Nursing Outlook, 34*(1), 16–19, 24.

Halcomb, R. (1979). *Women making it: Patterns and profiles of success.* New York: Atheneum.

Hall, R., & Sandler, B. R. (1983). Academic mentoring for women students and faculty: A new look at an old way to get ahead. In *Project on the status and education of women.* Washington, DC: Association of American Colleges.

Hamilton, E. M., Murray, M. K., Lindholm, L. H., & Myers, R. E. (1989). Effects of mentoring on job satisfaction, leadership behaviors, and job retention of new graduate nurses. *Journal of Nursing Staff Development, 5*(4), 159–165.

Hamilton, L., Vincent, L., Goode, R., Moorhouse, A., Worden, R. H., Jones, H., Close, M., & Dufour, S. (1990). Organizational support of the clinical nurse specialist role: A nursing research and professional development directorate. *Canadian Journal of Nursing Administration, 3*(3), 9–13.

Hanneman, S. K. (1996). Advancing nursing practice with a unit-based clinical expert. *Image: Journal of Nursing Scholarship, 28*(4), 331–337.

Hanson, C. M., & Hilde, E. (1989). Faculty mentorship: Support for nurse practitioner students and staff within the rural community health setting. *Journal of Community Health Nursing, 6*(2), 73–81.

Hardcastle, B. (1988). Spiritual connections: protégés' reflections on significant mentorships. *Theory into Practice, 27*(3), 201–208.

Hardy, L. K. (1983). *An exploration of the career histories of leading female nurses in England and Scotland.* Unpublished doctoral dissertation, University of Edinburgh, Scotland.

Hardy, L. K. (1986). *An exploration of the career histories of selected leading male nurses in England and Scotland.* Unpublished postdoctoral study, University of Lethbridge, Lethbridge, Alberta, Canada.

Haring-Hidore, M. (1991, April). *Mentoring mini-course.* Paper presented at the Annual Meeting of the American Educational Research Association, Chicago.

Hayes, E. (1994). Helping preceptors mentor the next generation of nurse practitioners. *Nurse Practitioner, 19*(6), 62–66.

Hayes, E., & Harrell, C. (1994). On being a mentor to nurse practitioner students: The preceptor-student relationship. *Nurse Practitioner Forum, 5*(4), 220–226.

Haynor, P. M. (1994). The coaching, precepting, and mentoring roles of the leader within an organizational setting. *Holistic Nurse Practitioner, 9*(1), 31–40.

Heinrich, K. T. (1992). Create a tradition: Teach nurses to share stories. *Journal of Nursing Education, 31*(3), 141–143.

Heinrich, K. T. (1995). Doctoral advisement relationships between women: On friendship and betrayal. *Journal of Higher Education, 66*(4), 447–469.

Heinrich, K. T., Rogers, A., Haley, R., & Taylor, A. (1995, October). *Doctoral study as heroic journey: The dialectic between the personal journey and creating community.* Paper presented at the Sixth Annual International Critical and Feminist Perspectives in Nursing Conference, Prout's Neck, ME.

Heinrich, K. T., & Scherr, M. W. (1994). Peer mentoring for reflective teaching: A model for nurses who teach. *Nurse Educator, 19*(4), 36–41.

Helgesen, S. (1990). *The female advantage: Women's ways of leadership.* New York: Doubleday.

Hennig, M. (1970). *Career development for women executives.* Unpublished doctoral dissertation, Harvard University, Boston, MA.

Hennig, M., & Jardim, A. (1977). *The managerial woman.* Garden City, NY: Doubleday.

Hinshaw, A. S. (1990). National center for nursing research: A commitment to excellence in science. In J. C. McCloskey & H. K. Grace (Eds.), *Current issues in nursing* (pp. 357–362). St. Louis: Mosby.

Hinshaw, A. S. (1992). Nursing research: Weaving the past and the future. In L. Aiken & C. Fagin (Eds.), *Charting nursing's future: Agenda for the 1990s* (pp. 485–503). Philadelphia: Lippincott.

Hinson, D. K. (1986). Identification of the mentor relationship in the career of a staff nurse (Master's thesis, University of Utah, 1986). *Master's Abstracts International, 25,* 199.

Hockenberry-Eaton, M., & Kline, N. (1995). Who is mentoring the nurse practitioner? *Journal of Pediatric Health Care, 9,* 94–95.

Hoffman, B. C. (1995). Mentoring of women and minority faculty and students. In E. Rubin (Ed.), *Building the workforce for a diverse society: Proceedings of the 3rd Congress of Health Profession Educators* (pp. 41–47). Washington, DC: Association of Academic Health Centers.

Holloran, S. D. (1989). Mentoring: The experience of nursing service executives (Doctoral dissertation, Boston University, 1989). *Dissertation Abstracts International, 50,* 3920B.

Holloran, S. D. (1993). Mentoring: The experience of nursing service executives. *Journal of Nursing Administration, 23*(2), 49–54.

Homer (1961). *The Odyssey.* (R. Fitzgerald, Trans.). New York: Doubleday.

Huang, C. A., & Lynch, J. (1995). *Mentoring: The tao of giving and receiving wisdom.* New York: HarperSanFrancisco.

Hughes, L. (1992). Faculty-student interactions and the student-perceived climate for caring. *Advances in Nursing Science, 14*(3), 60–71.

Hupcey, J. E. (1988). *The socialization process for master's level nurse practitioner students: Students' expectations of their future roles and the socialization factors which influence these role expectations.* Unpublished master's thesis, University of Washington, Seattle.

Hupcey, J. E. (1990). The socialization process of master's-level nurse practitioner students. *Journal of Nursing Education, 29*(5), 197–201.

Hyland-Hill, B. (1986). *Relationship between head nurse leadership effectiveness and presence or absence of a mentor.* Unpublished master's thesis, University of Washington, Seattle.

Jeruchim, J., & Shapiro, P. (1992). *Women, mentors, and success.* New York: Fawcett Columbine.

Joel, L. A. (1997). Charged to mentor. *American Journal of Nursing, 97*(2), 7.

Johantgen, M. E. (1985). *The prevalence and effects of helping relationships on staff nurses' career development.* Unpublished master's thesis, State University of New York, Buffalo.

Johnson, R. (1993). Nurse practitioner-patient discourse: Uncovering the voice of nursing in primary care practice. *Scholarly Inquiry for Nursing Practice: An International Journal, 7*(3), 143–157.

Johnsrud, L. K. (1991). Mentoring between academic women: The capacity for interdependence. *Initiatives, 54*(3), 7–17.

Jowers, L. T. , & Herr, K. (1990). A review of literature on mentor-protégé relationships. In G. M. Clayton & P. A. Baj (Eds.), *Review of Research in Nursing Education* (Vol. 3, pp. 49–77). New York: National League for Nursing.

Just, G. (1989). Mentors and self-reports of professionalism in hospital staff nurses. (Doctoral dissertation, New York University, 1989). *Dissertation Abstracts International, 51,* 664B.

Kanter, R. M. (1979). *Men and women in the corporation.* New York: Basic Books.

Kanter, R. M. (1984). *The change masters.* New York: Simon and Schuster.

Kanter, R. M. (1990). *When giants learn to dance.* New York: Simon and Schuster.

Kanter, R. M., & Stein, B. A. (1979). The gender pioneers: Women in an industrial sales force. In R. M. Kanter & B. A. Stein (Eds.), *Life in organizations.* New York: Basic Books.

Kavoosi, M. C., Elman, N. S., & Mauch, J. E. (1995). Faculty mentoring and administrative support in schools of nursing. *Journal of Nursing Education, 34*(9), 419–426.

Kegan, R. (1982). *The evolving self: Problem and process in human development.* Cambridge, MA: Harvard University Press.

Kelly, L. Y. (1978). Power guide—The mentor relationship. *Nursing Outlook, 26*(5), 339.

Kelly, L. Y. (1979). How to start a counterculture [End paper]. *Nursing Outlook, 28,* 149.

Kelly, L. Y. (1987). To touch tomorrow. *Nursing Outlook, 35,* 59.

Kerr, L. (1995). *Wisdom: A global ethic.* Vancouver: British Columbia: Cowichan Press.

Kim, M. J., & Felton, G. (1986). Research mentoring. *Journal of Professional Nursing, 2*(3), 142.

Kinsey, D. C. (1985). An updated group profile of contemporary influentials in American nursing (Doctoral dissertation, Lehigh University, 1985). *Dissertation Abstracts International, 46,* 1870B.

Kinsey, D. C. (1986). The new nurse influential. *Nursing Outlook, 34*(5), 238–240.

Kinsey, D. C. (1990). Mentorship and influence in nursing. *Nursing Management, 21*(5), 45–46.

Knebel, E. A. (1985). Profile of the mentor relationship in nursing service administration: A professional leadership development strategy (Doctoral dissertation, University of Houston, 1985). *Dissertation Abstracts International, 46,* 3258A.

Koerner, J., & McWhinney, W. (1995). *Uncommon wisdom: Experiences with remarkable people on the road towards mastery.* San Francisco: Center for Nursing Leadership.

Kotter, J. P. (1985). *Power and influence.* New York: Free Press.

Kram, K. E., & Isabella, L. A. (1985). Mentoring alternatives: The role of peer relationships in career development. *Academy of Management Journal, 28,* 110–132.

Krcmar, C. R. (1991). Organizational entry: The case of the clinical nurse specialist. *Clinical Nurse Specialist, 5,* 38–42.

Kremgold-Barrett, A. (1986). Women mentoring women in an academic nursing facility (Doctoral dissertation, Boston University, 1986). *Dissertation Abstracts International, 46,* 588B.

Kulig, J., & Thorpe, K. (1996). Teaching and learning needs of learning diverse post-RN students. *Canadian Journal of Nursing Research, 28*(2), 119–123.

Kundsin, R. B. (Ed.). (1974). *Women & success: The anatomy of achievement.* New York: William Morrow.

Lamb, G. S., & Stempel, J. E. (1994). Nursing case management from the client's view: Growing as insider-expert. *Nursing Outlook, 42*(1), 7–13.

Lamborn, M. L. (1991). Motivation and job satisfaction of deans of schools of nursing. *Journal of Professional Nursing, 7*(1), 33–40.

Lancaster, H. (1997, April 1). How women can find mentors in a world with few role models. *Wall Street Journal,* p. B1.

Larkin, D. M., & Zahourek, R. P. (1988). Therapeutic storytelling and metaphors. *Holistic Nursing Practice, 2*(3), 45–53.

Larson, B. A. (1980). *An exploratory study of the relationship of job satisfaction of nursing leaders in hospital settings who have had a mentor relationship and those who have not.* Unpublished master's thesis, University of Washington, Seattle.

Larson, B. A. (1986). Job satisfaction of nursing leaders with mentor relationships. *Nursing Administration Quarterly, 11*(1), 53–60.

Larson, O. M. (1994). Career aspirations to higher leadership positions of nurse faculty middle managers. *Journal of Professional Nursing, 10*(3), 147–153.

Leavitt, J., & Barry, C. (1993). Learning the ropes. In D. Mason, S. Talbott, & J. Leavitt (Eds.), *Policy and politics for nurses: Action and change in the workplace, government, organizations and community* (2nd ed.). (pp. 47–61). Philadelphia: Saunders.

Lee, C. A. (1988). Need motivation and mentorship experiences of national and state nursing leaders (Doctoral dissertation, Kansas State University, 1988). *Dissertation Abstracts International, 49,* 4754B.

Lee, P. (1997). North Carolina Association establishes mentoring program. *National Association of Women in Education News, 26*(1), 6, 17.

Leegard, M. (1993). The daily life ministry of the baptized believer. In *Grab the blessing.* Minneapolis: Sierra Book Club.

Leonard, G. (1992). *Mastery: The keys to success and long-term fulfillment.* New York: Penguin Books.

Levinson, D. (1996). *The seasons of a woman's life.* New York: Knopf.

Levinson, D. J., Darrow, C. N., Klein, E. B., Levinson, M. H., & McKee, B. (1978). *The seasons of a man's life.* New York: Knopf; paperback, Ballantine, 1979.

Linc, L. G., & Campbell, J. M. (1995). Role models for research. *Advanced Practice Nurse 2(2),* 19–21, 24.

Livingston, J. S. (1988). Pygmalion in management. *Harvard Business Review, 66*(5), 121–130.

Lough, M. E. (1986). Networking and working with a mentor: Keys to eliciting support for clinical support as a staff nurse. *Heart and Lung, 15,* 525–527.

Lumby, J. (1993). A feminist method. *Nursing New Zealand, 1(3),* 17–18.

Luna, G., & Cullen, D. L. (1995). *Empowering the faculty: Mentoring redirected and renewed.* ASHE-ERIC Higher Education Report No. 3. Washington, DC: George Washington University, Graduate School of Education and Human Development.

Lutz, S. (1995). The vanishing art of mentoring. *Modern Healthcare, 25,* 44–49.

Macey, J. C. (1985). A study of faculty protégé-mentor relationships as a method for faculty development in schools of nursing (Doctoral dissertation, Vanderbilt University, George Peabody College, 1985). *Dissertation Abstracts International, 46,* 1600A.

Madison, J. R. (1984). *A study to determine nurse administrators' perceptions of the mentoring relationship and its effect on their professional lives.* Unpublished master's thesis, University of Minnesota, Minneapolis.

Malone, B. L. (1981). Relationship of black female administrators' mentoring experience and career satisfaction (Doctoral dissertation, University of

Cincinnati, 1981). *Dissertation Abstracts International, 43,* 558B.

Marquis, B. L., & Huston, C. J. (1992). *Leadership roles and management function in nursing.* Philadelphia: Lippincott.

Martin, M. L., Tolleson, J., Lakey, K. I., & Moeller, E. (1995). VALOR students: A creative type of preceptorship. *Federal Practitioner, 12*(4), 47–50.

Mathews, K. R. (1988). Mentorship as a career advancement strategy in the United States Air Force nurse corps. (Master's thesis, University of New Mexico). *Master's Abstracts International, 27,* 99.

May, K. M., Meleis, A. I., & Winstead-Fry, P. (1982). Mentorship for scholarliness: Opportunities and dilemmas. *Nursing Outlook, 30*(1), 22–28.

McBride, A. B. (1994). President's message: A tribute to Jean E. Johnson. *Nursing Outlook, 42*(1), 39–42.

McCloskey, J. C., & Molen, M. T. (1987). Leadership in nursing. In J. J. Fitzpatrick, R. L. Taunton, & J. S. Benoliel (Eds.), *Annual review of nursing research, 5,* 177–201. New York: Springer Publishing.

McIntyre, D., Hagger, H., & Wilkin, M. (1993). *Mentoring: Perspectives on school-based teacher education.* London: Kogan Page.

Megel, M. E. (1985). New faculty in nursing: Socialization and the role of the mentor. *Journal of Nursing Education, 24*(7), 303–306.

Megel, M. E., Langston, N. F., & Creswell, J. W. (1988). Scholarly productivity: A survey of nursing faculty researchers. *Journal of Professional Nursing, 4*(1), 45–54.

Meleis, A. I. (1992). On the way to scholarship: From master's to doctorate. *Journal of Professional Nursing, 8*(6), 328–334.

Meleis, A. I., Hall, J. M., & Stevens, P. E. (1994). Scholarly caring in doctoral nursing education: Promoting diversity and collaborative mentorship. *Image: Journal of Nursing Scholarship, 26*(3), 177–180.

Merriam, S. (1983). Mentors and protégés. A critical review of the literature. *Adult Education Quarterly, 33*(3), 161–173.

Miller, J. B. (1976). *Toward a new psychology of women.* Boston: Beacon Press.

Miller, J. B. (1991). Women and power. In J. Jordan, A. Kaplan, J. B. Miller, I. Stiver, & J. Surrey (Eds.), *Women's growth in connection* (pp. 197–205). New York: Guilford Press.

Missirian, A. K. (1981). The process of mentoring in the career development of female managers. *Dissertation Abstracts International, 41,* 3654A. (University Microfilms No. 8101368, 189).

Moore, K. M. (1982). The role of mentors in developing leaders for academe. *Educational Record, 63*(1), 23–28.

Morales-Mann, E. T., & Higuchi, K. A. (1995). Transcultural mentoring: An experience in perspective transformation. *Journal of Nursing Education, 34*(6), 272–277.

Morrison, I. (1996). *The second curve: Managing the velocity of change.* New York: Ballantine Books.

Morrison, A., White, R., & VanVelsor, E. (1987). *Breaking the glass ceiling.* Reading, MA: Addison-Wesley.

Murray, M., & Owen, M. (1991). *Beyond the myths and magic of mentoring.* San Francisco: Jossey-Bass.

National Student Nurses Association. (1996). In support of the promotion, awareness, and development of mentorship programs. *Proceedings from NSNA Annual Convention—New Orleans, LA.* New York: Author.

Nelson, L. (1995). Mentoring toward a longed for life. In P. Munhall & V. Fitzsimmon (Eds.), *The emergence of women into the 21st century* (pp. 361–375). New York: National League for Nursing Press.

Noble, K. D. (1990). The female hero: A quest for healing and wholeness. *Women and Therapy, 9*(4), 3–18.

Noble, K. D. (1994). *The sound of a silver horn: Reclaiming the heroism in contemporary women's lives.* New York: Fawcett Columbine.

Noe, R. A. (1988a). An investigation of the determinants of successful assigned mentoring relationships. *Personnel Psychology, 41,* 457–479.

Noe, R. A. (1988b). Women and mentoring: A review and research agenda. *Academy of Management Review, 13*(1), 65–78.

Olson, R. K. (1984). An investigation of the selection process of mentor-protégé relationships among female nurse educators in college and university settings in the midwest (Doctoral dissertation, Saint Louis University, 1984). *Dissertation Abstracts International, 46,* 2259B.

Olson, R. K., & Connelly, L. M. (1995). Mentoring through predoctoral fellowships to enhance research productivity. *Journal of Professional Nursing, 11*(5), 270–275.

Olson, R. K., Gresley, R. S., & Heater, B. S. (1984). The effects of an undergraduate clinical internship on the self-concept and professional role mastery of baccalaureate nursing students. *Journal of Nursing Education, 23*(3), 105–108.

Olson, R. K., & Vance, C. N. (1993). *Mentorship in nursing: A collection of research abstracts with selected bibliographies—1977–1992.* Houston, TX: University of Texas Printing Services.

Olson, R. K., & Vance, C. N. (1998). Mentorship in nursing education. In K. A. Stevens (Ed.), *Review of research in nursing education, 8.* New York: National League for Nursing.

O'Neil, J. R. (1993). *The paradox of success: A book of renewal for leaders.* New York: G. P. Putnam's Sons.

O'Neil, J. R. (1995). *Success and your shadow.* Audiotape No.A260, Part l). Boulder, CO: Sounds True Audio.

O'Neil, J. R. (1996, July). Developing tomorrow's leaders today. *Keynote Address.* AACN Summer Seminar, Jackson Hole, WY.

Orth, C., Wilkinson, H., & Benfari, R. (1990). The manager's role as coach and mentor. *Journal of Nursing Administration, 29*(9), 11–15.

Pardue, S. (1983). The who-what-why of mentor teacher/graduate student relationships. *Journal of Nursing Education, 22*(9), 32–37.

Parks, S. D. (1992). *The university as a mentoring environment.* Indiana Office for Campus Ministries.

Personal Narrative Group. (1989). *Interpreting women's lives.* Bloomington: Indiana University Press.

Phillips, G. (1979). The peculiar intimacy of graduate study: A conservative view. *Communication Education, 28,* 339–345.

Pilette, P. C. (1980). Mentoring: An encounter of the leadership kind. *Nursing Leadership, 3*(2), 22–26.

Plato. (1968). *The Republic.* (A. Bloom, Trans.). New York: Basic Books.

Policinski, H. & Davidhizar, R. (1985). Mentoring the novice. *Nurse Education, 10*(3), 34–37.

Polkinghorne, D. E. (1988). *Narrative knowing and the human sciences.* Albany, NY: State University of New York Press.

Powell, S. R. (1990). Mentors in nursing in the university setting (Doctoral dissertation, University of Iowa, 1990). *Dissertation Abstracts International, 51,* 5810B.

Prestholdt, C. O. (1990). Modern mentoring: Strategies for developing contemporary nursing leadership. *Nursing Administration Quarterly, 15*(1), 20–27.

Price, C. A. (1997). Mentoring the mentoree is not a one-way street. *American Nephrology Nurses Association Journal, 24*(1), 10.

Princeton, J. C., & Gaspar, T. M. (1991). First-line nurse administrators in academe: How are they prepared, what do they do, and will they stay in their jobs? *Journal of Professional Nursing, 7*(2), 79–87.

Pyles, S. H. (1981). *Assessment related to cardiogenic shock: Discovery of nursing gestalt.* Unpublished master's thesis, Northwestern State University of Louisiana.

Pyles, S. H., & Stern, P. (1983). Discovery of nursing gestalt in critical care nursing: The importance of the gray gorilla syndrome. *Image: Journal of Nursing Scholarship, 15*(2), 51–57.

Ragins, B. R. (1989). Barriers to mentoring: The female manager's dilemma. *Human Relations, 42*(1), 1–22.

Ramsey, D. R., Thompson, J. C., & Brathwaite, H. (1994). Mentoring: A professional commitment. *Journal of the National Black Nurses' Association, 7*(1), 68–76.

Rankin, E. A. (1991). Mentor, mentee, mentoring: Building career development relationships. *Nursing Connections, 4*(4), 49–57.

Rawl, S. M. (1989). Nursing education administrators: Level of career development and mentoring (Doctoral dissertation, University of Illinois, Chicago, 1989). *Dissertation Abstracts International, 50,* 1857B.

Rawl, S. M., & Peterson, L. M. (1992). Nursing education administrators: Level of career development and mentoring. *Journal of Professional Nursing, 8*(3), 161–169.

Redmond, G. M. (1991). Life and career pathways of deans in nursing programs. *Journal of Professional Nursing, 7*(4), 228–238.

Redmond, G. M. (1995). "We don't make widgets here": Voices of chief nurse executives. *Journal of Nursing Administration, 25*(2), 63–69.

Redmond, S. P. (1990). Mentoring and cultural diversity in academic settings. *American Behavioral Scientist, 34*(2), 188–200.

Rempusheski, V. F. (1992). A researcher as resource, mentor, and preceptor. *Applied Nursing Research, 5*(2), 105–107.

Rew, L. (1996). Affirming cultural diversity: A pathways model for nursing faculty. *Journal of Nursing Education, 35*(7), 310–314.

Risco, K., & Hakos, L. (1992). Caring for the caregiver: The art of mentoring. *Pennsylvania Nurse, 4*, 16–17.

Rittman, M. R., & Sella, S. (1995). Storytelling: An innovative approach to staff development. *Journal of Nursing Staff Development, 11*(1), 15–19.

Roberts, S. J. (1983). Oppressed group behavior: Implications for nursing. *Advances in Nursing Science, 5*(7), 21–30.

Roche, G. (1979). Much ado about mentors. *Harvard Business Review, 57*(1), 14–16, 20, 24, 26–28.

Rogers, C. (1961). *On becoming a person.* Boston: Houghton Mifflin.

Rogers, C. (1978). *Carl Rogers on personal power.* London: Constable.

Rogers, J. L. (1988). New paradigm leadership: Integrating the female ethos. *Initiatives, 51*(4), 1–8.

Rosener, J. B. (1990). Ways women lead. *Harvard Business Review, 68*(6), 119–125.

Rosenow, A. M. (1981). The dilemma of achievement in nursing: A woman's profession (Doctoral dissertation, University of Chicago, 1981). *Dissertation Abstracts International, 43*, 2311B.

Rosenthal, R., & Jacobson, L. (1968). *Pygmalion in the classroom: Teacher expectation and pupils' intellectual development.* New York: Holt, Rinehart & Winston.

Rothman, B. K. (1984). Childbirth management and medical monopoly: Midwifery as (almost) a profession. *Journal of Nurse-Midwifery, 29*(5), 300–306.

Rzucidlo, S. E. (1992). The perceived role of mentoring in the career development of staff nurses in a clinical ladder system. (Master's thesis, Duquesne University, 1992). *Masters Abstracts International, 30*, 1299.

Sandelowski, M. (1991). Telling stories: Narrative approaches in qualitative research. *Image: Journal of Nursing Scholarship, 23*(3), 161–165.

Sandler, B. R. (1993, March 10). Women as mentors: Myths and commandments. *Chronicle of Higher Education*, p. B3.

Sandler, B. R., & Hoffman, E. (1992). *Teaching faculty members to be better teachers: A guide to equitable and effective classroom techniques.* Washington, DC: Association of American Colleges.

Schank, R. C. (1990). *Tell me a story: Narrative and intelligence.* Evanston, IL: Northwestern University Press.

Schneer, J. A., & Retiman, F. (1995). The impact of gender as managerial careers unfold. *Journal of Vocational Behavior, 47*, 290–315.

Schoolcraft, V. (1986). The relationship between mentoring and androgyny (Doctoral dissertation, University of Oklahoma, 1986). *Dissertation Abstracts International, 47,* 3681A.

Schoolcraft, V. (1995). Woman's work and being a mentor. In P. Munhall & V. Fitzsimons (Eds.), *The emergence of women into the 21st century* (pp. 337–348). New York: National League for Nursing Press.

Schorr, T. (1978). The lost art of mentorship. *American Journal of Nursing, 78,* 1873.

Schorr, T. (1979). Mentor remembered. *American Journal of Nursing, 79,* 65.

Schorr, T., & Zimmerman, A. (1988). *Making choices: Taking chances: Nurse leaders tell their stories.* St. Louis: Mosby.

Sealy, P. (1987). *Canadian master's students in nursing: Experiences with the mentor relationship.* Unpublished master's thesis, University of Western Ontario, London, Canada.

Senge, P. M. (1990). *The fifth discipline: The art and practice of the learning organization.* New York: Doubleday.

Senge, P. M., Kleiner, A., Roberts, C., Ross, R. B., & Smith, B. J. (1994). *The fifth discipline fieldbook.* New York: Doubleday.

Shapiro, E., Haseltine, F., & Rowe, M. (1978). Moving up: Role models, mentors, and the "patron system." *Sloan Management Review, 19*(3), 51–58.

Sheehy, G. (1976). *Passages: Predictable crises of adult life.* New York: Dutton.

Sheehy, G. (1995). *New passages: mapping your life across time.* New York: Ballantine.

Sheldon, A. (1990). A feminist perspective on women as mentors. *Career Planning and Adult Development, 6*(3), 16–20.

Short, J. D. (1994). *Mentoring among influential nurse administrators.* Unpublished doctoral dissertation, University of Alabama at Birmingham.

Short, J. D. (1997a). Profile of administrators of schools of nursing, Part 1: Resources for goal achievement. *Journal of Professional Nursing, 13*(1), 7–12.

Short, J. D. (1997b). Profile of administrators of schools of nursing, Part 2: Mentoring relationships and influence activities. *Journal of Professional Nursing, 13*(1), 13–18.

Sibley, P. (1991). Mentoring: Implications for the new research investigator. *Science Nursing, 8*(2), 53–54.

Slagle, J. (1986). The process of mentoring in nursing: A study of protégés' perceptions of the mentor-protégé relationship (Doctoral dissertation, Columbia University, Teachers College, 1986). *Dissertation Abstracts International, 47,* 2377B.

Spengler, C. D. (1982). Mentor-protégé relationships: A study of career development among female nurse doctorates. (Doctoral dissertation, University of Missouri, Columbia, 1982). *Dissertation Abstracts International, 44,* 2113B.

Stejskal, J. (1992). *Nursing and organizational culture at a Midwest hospital: A case study.* Unpublished doctoral dissertation, University of St. Thomas, St. Paul, MN.

Stewart, W. A. (1976). *A psychosocial study of the formation of the early adult life structure in women.* Unpublished doctoral dissertation, Columbia University, New York.

Stewart, B., & Krueger, L. (1996). An evolutionary concept analysis of mentoring in nursing. *Journal of Professional Nursing, 12*(5), 311–321.

Strachura, L. M., & Hoff, J. (1990). Toward achievement of mentoring for nurses. *Nursing Administration Quarterly, 15*(1), 56–62.

Super, D. E. (1957). *The psychology of careers.* New York: Harper.

Super, D. E. (1963). *Career development: Self-concept theory.* New York: Entrance Board.

Surrey, J. L. (1991). Relationship and empowerment. In J. V. Jordan, A. G. Kaplan, J. B. Miller, I. P. Stiver, & J. L. Surrey (Eds.), *Women's growth in connection* (pp. 162–180). New York: Guilford Press.

Swazey, J. P., & Anderson, M. S. (1996). *Mentors, advisors, and role models in graduate and professional education.* Washington, DC: Association of Academic Health Centers.

Tagg, M. I. (1986). Mentoring in nursing: A study of the career development of professional nurse faculty in selected colleges of nursing (Doctoral dissertation, Memphis State University, 1986). *Dissertation Abstracts International, 47,* 4826B.

Taylor, A. J. (1984). *Mentoring among nurse administrators.* Unpublished postmaster's study, British Columbia Institute of Technology, Vancouver, British Columbia, Canada.

Taylor, L. J. (1992). A survey of mentor relationships in academe. *Journal of Professional Nursing, 8*(1), 48–55.

Torsella, P. (1993). *The quantity, quality, and impact of mentoring relationships among nurse faculty in academe.* Unpublished doctoral dissertation, Widener University, Chester, PA.

Tully, E. (1994). Doing professionalism differently: A sociological analysis of midwifery autonomy. *Proceedings of the New Zealand College of Midwives Third National Conference,* Rotorua, New Zealand.

Turton, S., & Herriot, S. (1989). Mentoring psychiatric student nurses. *Nursing Times, 85*(36), 70–71.

United Nations, Department of Public Information. (1996). *Platform for action and the Beijing declaration.* New York: United Nations.

Vaillant, G. (1977). *Adaptation to life.* Boston: Little, Brown.

Vaillot, M. C. (1966). Existentialism: A philosophy of commitment. *American Journal of Nursing, 66,* 500–505.

Valadez, A. M., & Lund, C. A. (1993). Mentorship: Maslow and me. *Journal of Continuing Education in Nursing, 24*(6), 259–263.

Valverde, L. A. (1980). Development of ethnic researchers and the education of white researchers. *Educational Researcher, 9*(9), 16–20.

Vance, C. (1977). A group profile of contemporary influentials in American nursing (Doctoral dissertation, Teachers College, Columbia University, 1977). *Dissertation Abstracts International, 38,* 4734B.

Vance, C. (1979). Women leaders: Modern day heroines or societal deviants? *Image: Journal of Nursing Scholarship, 11*(2), 37–41.

Vance, C. (1982). The mentor connection. *Journal of Nursing Administration, 12*(4), 7–13.

Vance, C. (1986). The role of mentorship in the leadership development of nurse influentials. In W. A. Gray & M. M. Gray (Eds.), *Mentoring: Aid to excellence in career development, business, and the professions* (Vol. 2, pp. 177–184). Vancouver, British Columbia, Canada: International Association for Mentoring.

Vance, C. (1989–1990). Is there a mentor in your career future? *Imprint, 36*(5), 41–42.

Vance, C. (1992). Managing the politics of the workplace. *Imprint, 39*(1), 16, 18–19.

Vance, C. (1994). Mentoring for career success and satisfaction. *Australian Journal of Advanced Nursing, 11*(4), 3.

Vance, C. (1995). The teacher as mentor. *International Nurse, News and Views, 8*(2), 6.

Vance, C. (1996). What can we do to prepare our graduates? In *Bridging the gap between education and practice: How can new graduates leap the chasm from the classroom to a restructured health care system?* (pp. 1–13). New York: New York State Nurses Association.

Vance, C., & Olson, R. K. (1997). A new paradigm for mentorship. In Internatioanl Mentoring Association, *Diversity in mentoring.* (pp. 249–258). Kalamazoo, MI: Western Michigan University.

Vance, C., & Olson, R. K. (1991). Mentorship. In J. J. Fitzpatrick, R. L. Taunton, & A. K. Jacox (Eds.), *Annual Review of Nursing Research, 9* (pp. 175–200). New York: Springer.

van Manen, M. (1990). *Researching lived experience.* Albany, NY: State University of New York Press.

Vigen, K. L. (1992). The role of the dean from a liberal arts setting perspective. In R. Z. Booth (Ed.), *Executive development series 2: The dean's role in organizational assessment and development* (pp. 43–51). Washington, DC: American Association of Colleges of Nursing.

Vogt, R. B. (1985). The relationship of mentoring activity and career success of nursing faculty (Doctoral dissertation, Northern Illinois University, DeKalb, 1985). *Dissertation Abstracts International, 47,* 439A.

Walker, M. B. (1981). *Perceptions and opinions about the employment of women administrators in the community college system in Pennsylvania.* Unpublished doctoral dissertation, University of Pennsylvania, Philadelphia.

Walker, M. B. (1984). Mentors for nurses as women in academe: A role for leadership development. *Proceedings of the Second Conference on Research in Nursing Education.* San Francisco: C.S.E. Press.

Walker, M. B., & Frank, L. (1995). HIV / AIDS: An imperative for a new paradigm for caring. *Nursing & Health Care, 16*(6), 310–315.

Waters, C. M. (1996). Professional development in nursing research: A culturally diverse postdoctoral experience. *Image: Journal of Nursing Scholarship, 28*(1), 47–50.

Weekes, D. P. (1989). Mentor-protégé relationships: A critical element in affirmative action. *Nursing Outlook 37*(4), 156–157.

Werley, H. (1988). Harriet H. Werley. In T. M. Schorr & A. Zimmerman (Eds.), *Making choices: Taking chances: Nurse leaders tell their stories* (pp. 364–378). St. Louis: Mosby.

Werley, H., & Newcomb, B. (1983). The research mentor: A missing element in nursing? In N. L. Chaska (Ed.), *The nursing profession: A time to speak* (pp. 202–215. New York: McGraw-Hill.

Whatley, K. L. (1990). *Mentor-protégé relationships among female non-doctorally prepared nurses in one acute-care setting.* Unpublished master's thesis, University of Wisconsin, Eau Claire.

Wheatley, M. (1994). *Leadership and the new science: Learning about organizations from an orderly universe.* San Francisco: Berrett-Koehler.

Wheatley, M., & Hirsch, M. S. (1994). Five ways to leave your mentor. *MS,* (September), 106–108.

White, J. F. (1986). The perceived role of mentoring in the career development and success of academic nurse administrators (Doctoral dissertation, University of Pittsburgh, 1986) *Dissertation Abstracts International, 47,* 1947A.

White, J. F. (1988). The perceived role of mentoring in the career development and success of academic nurse administrators. *Journal of Professional Nursing, 4*(3), 178–185.

Williams, R. S. (1986). Relationship of mentoring by senior faculty to the productivity of junior faculty in the top twenty colleges of nursing in the United States (Doctoral dissertation, University of Michigan, 1986). *Dissertation Abstracts International, 47,* 3682A.

Williams, R., & Blackburn, R. T. (1988). Mentoring and junior faculty productivity. *Journal of Nursing Education, 27*(5), 204–209.

Witherell, C., & Noddings, N. (1991). *Stories lives tell: Narrative and dialogue in education.* New York: Teachers College Press.

Wocial, L. (1995). The role of mentors in promoting integrity and preventing scientific misconduct in nursing research. *Journal of Professional Nursing, 11*(5), 276–280.

Wold, J. (1993). *The effectiveness of a mentor program on student satisfaction and retention in a baccalaureate nursing program.* Unpublished doctoral dissertation, Georgia State University, Atlanta.

Wolf, N. (1993). *Fire with fire: The new female power and how it will change the 21st century.* New York: Random House.

Woodrow, P. (1994). Mentorship: Perceptions and pitfalls for nursing practice. *Journal of Advanced Nursing, 19,* 812–818.

Wright, C. M. (1987). Mentorship: A college contribution. *Research and Development in Higher Education, 10,* 215–220.

Wright, C. M. (1989). Implementation of nursing mentorship. *Research and Development in Higher Education, 11,* 104–109.

Wright, C. M. (1990). An innovation in a diploma program: The future potential of mentorship in nursing. *Nurse Education Today, 10,* 355–359.

Wright, C. M. (1992). *The development and testing of a conceptual model for the analysis of contemporary developmental relationships in nursing.* Unpublished doctoral dissertation, University of Wollongong, Australia.

Wright, C. M. (1993, May). Bureaucratic and nursing values: Prioritising the rules to be changed. *Proceedings from the Second National Forum of the Royal College of Nursing, Australia* (pp. 112–130). Melbourne, Australia: World Congress Center.

Wright, C. M. (1994a, July). *The construction and validation of the Wright Professional Value Inventory.* Paper presented at the Xi Omicron Conference, Hawkesbury, Australia.

Wright, C. M. (1994b, July). *Critical issues in nursing: A need for a change in the work structures in which nurses work.* Paper presented at the Sigma Theta Tau International and Royal College of Nursing Conference, Sydney, Australia.

Wright, C. M. (1995). Critical issues in nursing: The need for a change in the work environment. *Collegian, 2*(3), 5–13.

Yoder, L. H. (1990). Mentoring: A concept analysis. *Nursing Administration Quarterly, 15*(1), 9–19.

Yoder, L. H. (1992). A descriptive study of mentoring relationships experienced by army nurses in head nurse or nursing supervisor roles. *Military Medicine, 157*(10), 518–523.

Yoder, L. H. (1995). Staff nurses' career development relationships and self-reports of professionalism, job satisfaction, and intent to stay. *Nursing Research, 44*(5), 290–297.

Young, C. F. (1985). Women as protégés: The preceptual development of female doctoral students who have completed their initial mentor-protégé relationship (Doctoral dissertation, Syracuse University, 1985). *Dissertation Abstracts International, 47,* 1903A.

Zey, M. G. (1984). *The mentor connection.* Homewood, IL: Dow Jones-Irwin.

Zey, M. G. (1997). Development of a goal/success typology for corporate formal mentor programs. In International Mentoring Associations, *Diversity in mentoring,* (pp. 298–310). Kalamazoo, MI: Western Michigan University.

Zimmerman, L. M. (1983). Factors influencing career success of women in nursing (Doctoral dissertation, University of Nebraska, Lincoln, 1983). *Dissertation Abstracts International, 44,* 1065–1066B.

Index

Academic
  administrator, 139–140
  faculty, 136–139
  setting, mentoring in, 121–140
  students, 130–136
    graduate, 126–130
    undergraduate, 122–125
Advanced practice nursing,
    144–147
Advancement, as benefit of
    mentoring, 9
Affiliation
  significance of, 43–44
Affiliative relationship, competitive
    relationship, contrasted, 47
Alliances, formation of, 28, 31
American Academy of Nursing, 29
American Association of Colleges of
    Nursing, 162
American Nurses Association
    (A.N.A.) Ethnic/Racial
    Minority Doctoral Fellowship
    Program, 94
Androgynous style, evolution of, 6,
    43
Apprentice
  functioning as, 17
  subordinate relationship, 17
Athena, mythological source of
    mentoring concept, 101
Authoritarianism
  as mentoring barrier, 51
  significance of, 42

Bandura, A., 7
Barriers, to mentor connections,
    50–52
Belenky, M. F., 5
Benefits, of mentoring, 8–10

Bureaucratic
  organizations, 42
  style, command-and-control as, 43

Career
  advice, 29
  commitment to, 114
  mentoring throughout, 16–30
Career development, 15, 25
  mentoring for, 11–34
  models of, 13
  planning, 37
Career stages
  mentoring during, 14, 17–30
Career success, 3, 36
  as benefit of mentoring, 9
  mentoring link with, 16
Caring, in mentoring relationship, 31
Chain of influence, 10
Climate, of organization, 19, 23, 141
Clinical leader mentoring, 147–50
Clinical organizations, mentoring in,
    141
Coaching, as type of mentoring help,
    14, 68
Collaborative mentoring, 139
Colleague
  international, mentor relationships
    among, 175
  relationship with, 14, 17, 21
Collective mentorship, 158–167
Collegial, peer, mentoring, 3, 22
Collegiality, impact of, 114
Competition
  effect of, 44
  evolution from, 111
  males and, 86
Competitive relationship, affiliative
    relationship, contrasted, 47

Conflict resolution, 135
Cooperation, movement towards, 111
Cronyism, 72
Cross-cultural mentoring, 171–203
Cross-gender mentor relationships, 139
Culture of learning, future development of, 207
Cyclic mentoring, ongoing mentoring, contrasted, 46–47

Dalton, G., 16
Development, life-career, stages of, 14
Developmental
    models, 11–13
    relationship, mentoring as, 3, 100–104
Dissenter perspective, 70–74, 100–104
Diversity, racial, mentoring and, 58–60

Empathetic understanding, importance of, 98
Empowerment, 43
    power, contrasted, 47–48
Erikson, E., 7
Exchange students, mentor relationships, 174–175
Exclusion, inclusion, contrasted, 44–45
Executive
    nurse as, 27
    woman as, 36
Executive development, mentorship and, 163–164
Expectation effect, 124
    significance of, 4
Expectations, in peer mentorship, 91
Expert-to-novice relationship, peer-to-peer relationship, contrasted, 46

Faculty, in mentoring relationships, 40, 136–139
    research productivity and, 23
Female
    ethos, 43
    mentoring, 31, 48–50. See also Women
Formal mentoring, 107–113, 130
Friendship, development of, from mentoring, 22

Future developments, in mentoring, 206–207

Gender, mentoring and, 31, 35–52
Generational effect, creation of, in mentoring, 24, 50
Gilligan, C., 5, 12
Global mentoring, 171–203
    collaborative nature of, 176–178
Graduate student mentoring, 126–130
Group mentorship, 158–167
Guidance, provision of, 29, 107

Hazing
    peer mentorship and, 93
    professional, as mentoring barrier, 51
Head nurse, mentorship, leadership, 148
Helgesen, S., 5
Hierarchy, 75, 86
    competition and, 44

Inclusion
    exclusion, contrasted, 44–45
    process of, 30, 43
    significance of, 31
Influence
    chain of, 10
    development of, 31
    in mentoring, 6
Informal mentor relationship, 107–113
Innovation, in mentoring, 207
Interactional process, in mentoring, 87–89, 102
International
    colleagues, mentor relationships among, 175
    educational program development, mentoring for, 172–173
    mentoring
        Australia, 196–199
        China, 178–185
        India, 192–196
        Italy, 199–201
        New Zealand, 185–188
        Philippines, 188–191
        Russia, 176–178, 201–203

students, mentoring of, 173–174
Invisible college, 3
Isolation, as mentoring barrier, 50, 51
"I-thou" relationship, influence of, 146

Job
    dissatisfaction with mentoring, 19
    satisfaction with mentoring, 16

Kellogg Foundation, 158–160

Leadership, 5, 9
    behaviors of, 143
    development of, 5, 15, 38, 162–167,
    interactive-inclusive style, 43
    model, 43
    roles, as benefit of mentoring, 9
    significance of, 31
    succession, 109
Learning
    culture of, future development of, 207
    mutual, in mentoring, 85
Learning organization, 109
Legacy, of mentoring, development of,
        207
Levinson, D. J., 5
Levinson, M. H., 5
Life-career development, stages of, 14
Limited mentoring, long-term
        mentoring, contrasted, 46
Long-distance leaders, 29

Magnet nursing department,
        mentorship in, 112–113
Manager, as mentor, 110
Maps, developmental, 12
Master-apprentice, 142
Mentor, in Greek mythology, 4, 101
Mentor emeritus, as type of mentoring
        help, 14
Mentor-protégé relationship, 17
Mentor relationship, nature of, 7–8
Mentoring
    barriers to, 50–52
    benefits of, 8–10
    commandments of, 165
    commitment, 22
    constraints, 51
    continuum, 38

formal, 107–113, 130
Future developments, 206–207
informal, 107–113
throughout career, 16–30
traditional, 22
types of, 14
    intellectual-guide, 14
    mentor emeritus, 14
    parent-sponsor, 14
    peer-colleague, 14
    promotor-coach, 14
    visionary-idealist, 14
    world views, 42–48
Midwives, mentoring of, 89
    New Zealand, 185–188
Modeling, 8
Mutuality, 5, 44
    in mentoring relationship, 85, 109
Mythological sources of mentoring
        concept
    Athena, 4, 101
    Hercules, 4
    Mentor, 4
    Odysseus, 4, 101

Narratives, use of in mentoring, 55
National Association of Women, 110
National Student Nurses Association, 122
Nature of relationship, in mentoring,
        7–8
Negotiation, in mentor relationship,
        107–17
Neophyte workers, students,
        socialization of, 109
Network
    old boys, 35, 71
    old girls, 160–162
    Philippine Nurses, 188–191
Networking, mentoring and, 15, 28,
        30–34, 35, 37
New mentorship, 7
    traditional mentorship, contrasted, 45
Nightingale, Florence, 6, 97
Nontraditional mentors, 22, 48–49, 51
Nurse
    executives, 27
    influential, 28–31, 50, 139–141
    mentoring to nurse, 35–52
    midwives. *See* Midwives

Nursing research, mentoring and,
　　151–157, 178–182
Nursing science, advances in, mentor
　　and, 151–153

Ongoing mentoring, cyclic mentoring,
　　contrasted, 46–47
Oppressed mentality, as mentoring
　　barrier, 50
Oppressed persons, mentoring and,
　　84, 135
Organizational climate, 19, 23, 141
Organizations, bureaucratic, 42

Paradigm
　　life-career stages, table, 14
　　mentoring, 42–48
Patriarchal style, effect of, 42, 44
Patron-protégé relationship, 32, 36
Peer-colleague, mentoring relation-
　　ship, 14, 17, 22
Peer mentorship, 89–93
　　expectations in, 91
　　influences in, 92
　　nontraditional, 22
Pew Charitable Trusts Foundation,
　　166
Political mentoring, 32, 160
Political support, without mentor net-
　　work, 35
Power
　　development of, 31
　　empowerment, contrasted, 47–48
　　significance of, 31
Practice setting, mentoring in, 141–150
Preceptorships, 25
Professional constraints, to
　　mentoring, 51
Professional development, of woman,
　　29, 38
Prophecy, self-fulfilling, from
　　influence of expectation, 73, 125
Protégé, mentor relationship, 5, 8, 17,
　　36, 60–66
　　maximizing role of, 82

Queen-bee syndrome, as mentoring
　　barrier, 19, 50, 58, 73

Racial diversity, mentoring and, 58–60
Racism, as obstacle to mentoring, 87
Reciprocity, in relationship, 48, 74
Relational capacities, in nursing, men-
　　toring and, 97–100
Relationship
　　developmental, 3
　　mentoring, nature of, 7–8
Research
　　development, mentoring for,
　　　151–157
　　nursing, mentoring and, 155–156
　　productivity of, with faculty, in
　　　mentoring relationship, 23
Responsibility, of mentoring, 93–97
Robert Wood Johnson Foundation, 75
Rogers, Carl, 98
Role, clarity of, 22, 23
Role-modeling, 5, 6, 9, 12, 29, 30–34,
　　37, 79
Role socialization, in mentoring
　　relationship, 23

Satisfaction, mentoring link with, 16
Scholarship, mentoring for, 151–157
Science, nursing, advances in,
　　mentor and, 151–153
Self-development, mentoring for,
　　11–34
Self-esteem, as benefit of mentoring, 9
Self-fulfilling prophecy, from
　　influence of expectation, 73, 125
Senge, P. M., 15
Sex-role, influence of, 37
Sigma Theta Tau International, 111
Socialization
　　importance of process, 12
　　of neophyte workers, students, 109
　　process of, 19
　　role, 23
Sponsorship, in mentoring
　　relationship, 14, 17, 22, 28, 31, 32
Storytelling
　　sense of history from, 28, 55
Success, in career
　　mentoring link with, 3, 16
Succession, in leadership, as benefit of
　　mentoring, 9

Super, D. E., model vocational life stages of, 13

Team players, 51
Traditional mentorship, new mentorship, contrasted, 45
Transformation, wisdomkeeper and, 80
Transition points, in career, personal life, 22
Troubleshooting, mentor relationship, 115–16

Undergraduate student mentoring, 122–125

Understanding, empathetic, importance of, 98
"Unintentional" mentors, 108–109

Values, in mentoring, 43
Voice, through mentoring, 7, 37

Web, strategy of, 31
Wisdom, mentorship and, 77–78
Wisdomkeeper
  becoming, 83–104
  contributions of, 78–79
  selection of, 79–82
Women, mentoring of women, 35–52
World views, of mentoring, 42–48

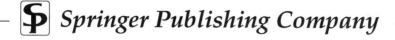 **Springer Publishing Company**

Writing and Getting Published
A Primer for Nurses
Barbara Stevens Barnum, RN, PhD, FAAN

This book, by one of nursing's most accomplished authors, is a step-by-step guide to developing professional writing skills and navigating the publication process. It includes pointers on structuring one's writing, avoiding common mistakes, making a term paper or dissertation publishable, writing query letters and book proposals, and finding and working with a publisher. The ability to communicate effectively in writing is an important tool for sharing knowledge and expertise, and for advancing a career. This concise guide demystifies the skills and procedures necessary to make this happen.

Contents:

Part I. Writing the Article • Finding the Right Topic • Writing the Article • Avoiding Common Mistakes • It's a Great Term Paper: Why Don't You Get it Published? • Publication Options: Sending Your Article to the Right Journal • What about a Query Letter? • Submitting Articles: Getting the Procedures Right • When Your Article Reaches the Journal

Part II. Writing the Book • How Book Writing Differs from Article Writing • The Edited or Coauthored Book • It's a Great Dissertation, But is it a Book? • Producing the Book Prospectus • Finding and Working with a Publisher

Part III. Special Issues • Writing with Colleagues • Writing from Research • Writing about Work Instruments

Appendices • Appendix A: List of Nursing Journals • Appendix B: List of Nursing Book Publishers • Appendix C: Additional Writing Resources

1995   216pp   0-8261-8690-4   hardcover

536 Broadway, New York, NY 10012-3955 • (212) 431-4370 • Fax (212) 941-7842

Ｓ *Springer Publishing Company*

The Role of The Preceptor
A Guide for Nurse Educators and Clinicians

Jean Pieri Flynn, EdD, RN

A practical "how to" guide for nursing faculty and administrators who want to set up preceptor programs, to guide student clinical experiences, or to help orient novice practitioners to the practice setting.

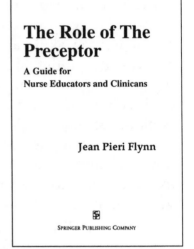

The Role of The
Preceptor
A Guide for
Nurse Educators and Clinicians

Jean Pieri Flynn

Ｓ
SPRINGER PUBLISHING COMPANY

The heart of the book is the description of two model preceptor programs — one at a university, and one in a large, urban medical center — illustrating how these programs can and do work in real life. Included are sample forms and procedures that can be adapted to your own institution's requirements.

Contents:

- Precepting, Not Mentoring or Teaching: Vive la Difference,
  B. Barnum
- Adult Learning Concepts Important to Precepting,
  M.J. Manley
- A Model Preceptor Program for Student Nurses, *A. O'Mara*
- An On-the-Job Preceptor Model for Newly Hired Nurses,
  J. Mackin and *K. Studva*
- Beyond Preceptorship: Internship and Externships, Fellow-ships / Apprenticeships and Mentorships, *Anne Belcher*

1997   152pp   0-8261-9460-5   hardcover

536 Broadway, New York, NY 10012-3955 • (212) 431-4370 • Fax (212) 941-7842

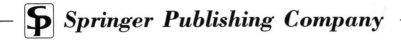

Springer Publishing Company

Successful Grant Writing
Strategies for Health and Human Service Professionals

Laura N. Gitlin, PhD and **Kevin J. Lyons,** PhD

This book guides the reader through the language and basic components of grantmanship. It illustrates how to develop ideas for funding, write the sections of a proposal, organize different types of project structures, and finally, how to understand the review process.

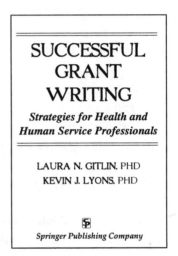

SUCCESSFUL
GRANT
WRITING

*Strategies for Health and
Human Service Professionals*

LAURA N. GITLIN, PHD
KEVIN J. LYONS, PHD

Springer Publishing Company

Each chapter describes a specific aspect of grantmanship and suggests innovative strategies to implement the information that is presented. The appendices contain helpful materials, such as a list of key acronyms, examples of timelines and sample budget sheets. The strategies in this volume are beneficial to individuals and departments in academic, clinical, or community-based settings.

Partial Contents:
- Becoming Familiar with Funding Sources
- Developing Your Ideas for Funding
- Learning about Your Institution
- Common Sections of Proposals
- Preparing a Budget
- Technical Considerations
- Strategies for Effective Writing
- Understanding the Process of Collaboration
- Understanding the Review Process

1996   235pp   0-8261-9260-2   hardcover

536 Broadway, New York, NY 10012-3955 • (212) 431-4370 • Fax (212) 941-7842

⑤ *Springer Publishing Company*

A Nurse's Guide to Public Speaking

Barry Jay Kaplan, MFA

Tailored to the specific needs of nurses, this information-packed guide is designed to help develop public speaking skills. The author outlines concrete steps for preparing and delivering a speech, including how to:

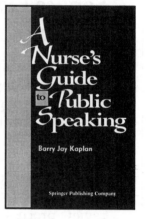

- Organize the speech
- Assess the room and audience
- Perform relaxation exercises before the speech
- Break the fear barrier

Nurses are called upon daily to use speaking skills in a wide variety of situations: in conferences, staff meetings, teaching, addressing patient and community groups. This book refers to these and other situations with practical suggestions on how to speak concisely and effectively. Honest and illuminating quotations from prominent nurses on their experiences as speakers are presented throughout the book.

Contents:

- What to Know Before You Make Your Speech
- Prepare Your Speech
- Prepare Yourself
- Breaking the Fear Barrier
- Making the Speech
- Who Owns the Speech
- Transforming a Speech into a Paper, a Paper into a Speech
- Other Forms of Oral Communication

1997   128pp   0-8261-9590-3   softcover

536 Broadway, New York, NY 10012-3955 • (212) 431-4370 • Fax (212) 941-7842